Vagus Nerve

How to Stimulate Vagus Nerve
With 4-week

*(Psychological and Emotional Manipulation With
Self-help Exercises for Trauma Depression)*

Dennis Campbell

Published By **Elena Holly**

Dennis Campbell

All Rights Reserved

Vagus Nerve: How to Stimulate Vagus Nerve With 4-week (Psychological and Emotional Manipulation With Self-help Exercises for Trauma Depression)

ISBN 978-1-7751012-5-3

No part of this guidebook shall be reproduced in any form without permission in writing from the publisher except in the case of brief quotations embodied in critical articles or reviews.

Legal & Disclaimer

The information contained in this book is not designed to replace or take the place of any form of medicine or professional medical advice. The information in this book has been provided for educational & entertainment purposes only.

The information contained in this book has been compiled from sources deemed reliable, and it is accurate to the best of the Author's knowledge; however, the Author cannot guarantee its accuracy and validity and cannot be held liable for any errors or omissions. Changes are periodically made to this book. You must consult your doctor or get professional medical advice before using any of the suggested remedies, techniques, or information in this book.

Table Of Contents

Chapter 1: Anatomy And Physiology

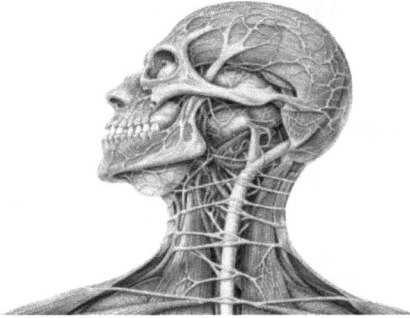

The vagus nerve is one of the longest and most complex nerves inside the frame. It is a cranial nerve that originates inside the brainstem and extends right all of the way right down to the stomach, passing through numerous organs and tissues alongside the way. The word "vagus" way "wandering" in Latin, that is becoming because of the reality the nerve has a meandering route at a few level inside the body.

The vagus nerve is answerable for a good sized form of abilities, on the facet of regulating coronary coronary coronary heart rate, breathing, digestion, and immune reaction. It is also concerned in sensory and motor talents of the top and neck, which incorporates flavor, speech, and facial expressions.

Due to its large obtain and severa talents, the vagus nerve has been the situation of a high-quality deal studies in modern day years. Scientists have discovered that stimulating the vagus nerve may have recuperation effects on an entire lot of conditions, which includes melancholy, epilepsy, and inflammatory illnesses.

In the subsequent sections, we're able to find out the anatomy and body shape of the vagus nerve in greater detail, collectively with its form, feature, and function in the frame.

The Structure of the Vagus Nerve

The vagus nerve is a paired nerve that originates inside the brainstem and extends down via the neck and chest to the belly. The nerve is crafted from every sensory and motor fibers, which means that that it could every experience and manipulate numerous functions inside the frame.

The vagus nerve is cut up into essential branches, the left and right vagus nerves. Each branch has severa smaller branches that innervate great organs and tissues in the body. The left vagus nerve basically innervates the coronary heart and lungs, while the right vagus nerve generally innervates the digestive tool.

The vagus nerve is composed of every myelinated and unmyelinated fibers. Myelinated fibers are blanketed in a fatty substance called myelin, which permits to rush up the transmission of nerve impulses. Unmyelinated fibers, however, are not blanketed in myelin and transmit nerve impulses more slowly.

The vagus nerve additionally consists of each afferent and efferent fibers. Afferent fibers carry sensory records from the organs and tissues over again to the thoughts, while efferent fibers deliver motor signs from the thoughts to the organs and tissues.

Overall, the form of the vagus nerve is fairly complicated and plays a vital characteristic in regulating many one-of-a-type physical capabilities. Understanding the anatomy of the vagus nerve is important for understanding how it talents and the manner it can be centered for therapeutic interventions.

The Function of the Vagus Nerve

The vagus nerve is a big element of the parasympathetic tense device, that is answerable for regulating the body's rest and digest reaction. The nerve originates within the medulla oblongata of the brainstem and extends down through the neck and chest, branching out to diverse organs and tissues at some point of the frame.

One of the primary abilities of the vagus nerve is to control the coronary coronary heart rate and rhythm. It does this with the useful resource of sending indicators to the sinoatrial node, the natural pacemaker of the coronary coronary heart, to slow down or accelerate the heart beat as needed. This is why deep respiration sporting sports and specific relaxation techniques that stimulate the vagus nerve may be powerful in reducing stress and tension.

The vagus nerve moreover plays a characteristic in digestion, stimulating the producing of digestive enzymes and growing blood go with the flow to the digestive tract. It moreover permits to alter bowel moves and prevent constipation.

In addition, the vagus nerve is concerned within the law of breathing function, controlling the fee and intensity of breathing. It also plays a function inside the immune device, assisting to reduce infection and sell restoration.

Overall, the vagus nerve is a important trouble of the frame's autonomic worried system, assisting to alter many crucial capabilities and preserve everyday fitness and nicely-being. Understanding its function and position in the body is critical for all and sundry interested by optimizing their health and well-being.

The Role of the Vagus Nerve in the Body

The vagus nerve is vital to the frame's autonomic frightened device, which controls among the bodily competencies that we do not consciously think about, along side heart fee, digestion, and respiratory.

One of the maximum vital roles of the vagus nerve is in regulating the coronary coronary heart charge. The nerve permits to sluggish down the coronary coronary heart fee whilst we're at relaxation, which enables to maintain strength and decrease pressure on the coronary heart. It additionally allows to modify blood stress via controlling the diameter of blood vessels.

The vagus nerve additionally performs a key function in digestion. It allows to stimulate the manufacturing of belly acid and digestive enzymes, which might be crucial for breaking down food. It moreover permits to adjust the motion of meals thru the digestive tract, ensuring that vitamins are absorbed successfully.

In addition to its function in regulating the coronary coronary heart and digestion, the vagus nerve additionally influences the immune system. It facilitates to lessen infection in the body, that is important for preventing continual illnesses together with arthritis and coronary coronary coronary heart sickness.

Overall, the vagus nerve is a primary part of the body's autonomic involved system, regulating many essential physical capabilities. Understanding the characteristic of the vagus nerve can help us to better apprehend our our our bodies.

Disorders and Conditions Related to the Vagus Nerve

Dysfunction of the vagus nerve is related to severa health conditions. Here are a number of the maximum commonplace problems linked to horrible functioning of the vagus nerve:

1. Gastroparesis: This is a situation wherein the belly takes too long to drain its contents. The vagus nerve controls the muscle groups that skip meals through the digestive machine. Damage to the nerve can bring about gastroparesis.

2. Heart arrhythmias: The vagus nerve lets in adjust the coronary heart price. Damage to the nerve can cause ordinary heartbeats or arrhythmias.

3. Epilepsy: Vagus nerve stimulation has been used as a remedy for epilepsy. It is assumed that the stimulation of the nerve can assist lessen the frequency and severity of seizures.

four. Depression and tension: The vagus nerve is involved in the law of temper and emotions. Studies have proven that stimulation of the nerve can help alleviate symptoms of depression and tension.

5. Inflammatory bowel illness: The vagus nerve allows adjust infection inside the body. Inflammatory bowel diseases, inclusive of Crohn's illness and ulcerative colitis, can be exacerbated by means of using harm to the nerve.

6. Obesity: The vagus nerve is involved in the law of urge for food and satiety. Damage to the nerve can bring about overeating and weight issues.

It's critical to phrase that no longer all issues and situations related to the vagus nerve are because of harm to the nerve. In a few times, the nerve may be functioning nicely, however different factors may be inflicting the symptoms. Nonetheless, knowledge the feature of the vagus nerve in those conditions can help healthcare specialists increase effective treatments and restoration methods.

three. Functions of the Vagus Nerve

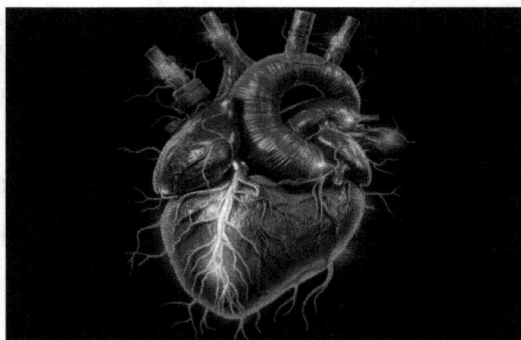

the Vagus Nerve and Its Importance

The vagus nerve is one of the maximum essential nerves within the frame, answerable for a significant kind of capabilities which may be critical to our ordinary health and nicely-being.

The vagus nerve is a part of the parasympathetic worried gadget, this is accountable for the "relaxation and digest" reaction inside the frame. This manner that once the vagus nerve is activated, it permits to slow down our coronary coronary heart charge, lower our blood pressure, and boom digestive hobby. It moreover performs a incredible detail in regulating our breathing and controlling contamination throughout the frame.

In addition to its function inside the parasympathetic fearful device, the vagus nerve is also cautiously associated with our emotional and intellectual fitness. Studies have tested that stimulating the vagus nerve can assist to reduce signs and symptoms of melancholy and tension, and may even decorate cognitive characteristic and reminiscence.

Given its huge kind of skills and significance to our standard fitness, it is clean that the vagus nerve is a subject that deserves our hobby and expertise. In the following sections, we are able to discover the severa approaches wherein this nerve influences our our bodies and minds, and the way we're able to harness its strength to decorate our fitness and well-being.

The Role of the Vagus Nerve in the Parasympathetic Nervous System

The parasympathetic disturbing device is chargeable for regulating relaxation and digestive interest. It allows to slow down the coronary coronary heart rate, reduce blood stress, and boom digestive hobby. The vagus nerve is the primary nerve accountable for transmitting parasympathetic alerts to the organs.

When the body is in a kingdom of strain or tension, the sympathetic nervous gadget is activated, primary to the "fight or flight" reaction. However, even as the chance has exceeded, the parasympathetic involved tool takes over to assist the frame pass lower back to a state of calm.

The vagus nerve allows to slow down the heart price and reduce blood pressure, which in turn allows to reduce emotions of anxiety and stress. It additionally stimulates the digestive system, growing the manufacturing of digestive enzymes and promoting the absorption of nutrients. This is why human beings often experience a feel of calm and relaxation after an fantastic meal.

In addition to its characteristic within the parasympathetic frightened system, the vagus nerve moreover performs a role in regulating infection within the body. It allows to reduce the producing of seasoned-inflammatory cytokines, that can make a contribution to a number of fitness troubles, along with chronic ache, autoimmune issues, and melancholy.

Overall, the vagus nerve is an vital organ of the parasympathetic concerned gadget, assisting to modify the frame's response to strain and sell relaxation and digestion.

The Vagus Nerve and Its Impact on Digestion

The vagus nerve is accountable for controlling the motion of meals via the digestive tract and the secretion of digestive juices. When the vagus nerve is activated, it stimulates the release of digestive enzymes and will growth blood go along with the flow to the digestive organs, which complements the absorption of vitamins from food.

Moreover, the vagus nerve is also involved in the law of urge for meals and satiety. It sends indicators to the mind to suggest while the stomach is whole, which lets in to save you overeating and maintain a healthy weight. In addition, the vagus nerve influences the secretion of hormones that manipulate hunger and metabolism, which includes ghrelin and leptin.

However, at the same time as the vagus nerve is not functioning properly, it could bring about digestive issues which consist of gastroparesis, in which the stomach takes too lengthy to drain its contents, and irritable bowel syndrome (IBS), which motives stomach ache, bloating, and modifications in bowel behavior. In such cases, stimulating the vagus nerve via techniques collectively with deep breathing, meditation, and acupuncture can help to relieve symptoms and symptoms and enhance digestion.

The Vagus Nerve and Its Connection to the Heart

The vagus nerve is capable for slowing down the coronary coronary coronary heart charge and lowering blood pressure, which allows to maintain a wholesome cardiovascular tool. The vagus nerve achieves this through using using releasing a neurotransmitter known as acetylcholine, which acts on the coronary coronary coronary heart's pacemaker cells to sluggish down the coronary coronary coronary heart price.

In addition to regulating coronary heart price, the vagus nerve moreover facilitates to keep coronary coronary coronary heart rhythm. It does this by modulating the electric hobby of the heart, that is critical for proper coronary coronary heart function. When the vagus nerve is activated, it may lessen the chance of arrhythmias, which may be uncommon coronary coronary heart rhythms that can be life-threatening.

Research has moreover showed that the vagus nerve also can have a shielding effect at the heart. Studies have located that humans with better vagal tone, it really is a degree of vagus nerve pastime, have a decrease threat of developing cardiovascular disease. This is due to the reality the vagus nerve lets in to lessen contamination, that may be a extremely good contributor to coronary heart sickness.

Overall, the vagus nerve performs a vital characteristic in keeping a healthy coronary coronary heart. By regulating coronary coronary heart price, rhythm, and infection, it permits to lessen the danger of cardiovascular disorder and promote normal cardiovascular fitness.

Chapter 2: Stimulation

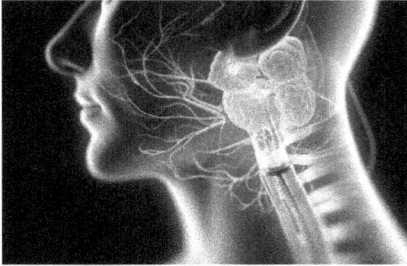

Understanding Vagus Nerve Stimulation

Vagus nerve stimulation (VNS) is a systematic way that includes the usage of electric impulses to stimulate the vagus nerve.

The method consists of the implantation of a small tool, similar to a pacemaker, under the pores and pores and skin in the chest location. The device is established to the vagus nerve thru a wire, and it sends electric powered impulses to the nerve at ordinary intervals. The frequency and depth of the impulses can be adjusted by way of the use of the use of a healthcare expert to healthy the affected individual's needs.

The cause of VNS is to spark off the vagus nerve, that would assist regulate diverse physical capabilities. It is robust in treating epilepsy, despair, and persistent ache, among one-of-a-kind situations. The actual mechanism by way of the usage of which VNS works isn't absolutely understood, but it's miles believed to contain the modulation of neurotransmitters inside the mind and the law of inflammation inside the frame.

VNS is normally taken into consideration safe, but like numerous scientific approach, it does supply a few risks. These include infection, bleeding, and harm to the nerve or surrounding tissues. Patients who undergo VNS need to be cautiously monitored with the useful resource of a healthcare expert to ensure that the tool is functioning properly and that any capability headaches are identified and addressed right away.

The Benefits of Vagus Nerve Stimulation

Vagus nerve stimulation has been placed to have a large kind of blessings for every physical and intellectual health. One of the maximum huge benefits of VNS is its functionality to lessen infection in the frame. Inflammation is a herbal reaction to injury or infection, however at the same time as it becomes chronic, it may result in a set of health troubles, which incorporates coronary heart illness, diabetes, or even most cancers. VNS has been shown to reduce infection with the aid of regulating the immune gadget and lowering the producing of pro-inflammatory cytokines.

Another benefit of VNS is its capability to enhance temper and decrease signs and symptoms of depression and tension. The vagus nerve is set up to the brain's limbic device, it sincerely is liable for regulating emotions. By stimulating the vagus nerve, VNS can assist alter temper and decrease signs and symptoms of depression and tension. Studies have confirmed that VNS may be an effective remedy for depression, even in patients who've no longer responded to traditional antidepressant medicinal tablets.

VNS has also been determined to have blessings for a whole lot of various situations, together with epilepsy, continual pain, and migraines. In sufferers with epilepsy, VNS can help lessen the frequency and severity of seizures. In patients with chronic pain, VNS can help lessen pain degrees and decorate best of lifestyles. In patients with migraines, VNS can assist reduce the frequency and intensity of headaches.

Different Methods of Vagus Nerve Stimulation

Several amazing techniques of vagus nerve stimulation were evolved through the years. Each method has its specific benefits and downsides, and the exceptional technique for you may depend on your person wishes and alternatives.

One of the maximum commonplace strategies of vagus nerve stimulation is through using an implanted device. This tool is surgically implanted underneath the pores and skin of the chest and is established to a twine that runs as plenty due to the fact the vagus nerve within the neck. The tool ensures electric powered impulses to the nerve, that could help to modify quite a few bodily skills.

Another method of vagus nerve stimulation is thru using a non-invasive device this is located on the pores and pores and skin of the neck. This device uses a small electric cutting-edge-day to stimulate the nerve and may be utilized in severa settings, collectively with at home or in a scientific workplace.

Several one of a kind strategies of vagus nerve stimulation are presently being superior and tested. For example, some researchers are exploring the usage of transcutaneous vagus nerve stimulation (TVNS), which includes using a small electric current done to the pores and skin overlying the nerve.

Overall, the tremendous methods of vagus nerve stimulation offer various alternatives for human beings trying to find to enhance their health and nicely-being. Whether you pick out an implanted tool or a non-invasive method, this treatment has the capability to make a extensive difference for your life.

Vagus Nerve Stimulation for Mental Health

Vagus nerve stimulation is an effective treatment for a number of intellectual fitness conditions. By stimulating the vagus nerve, this is liable for regulating the body's parasympathetic frightened tool, VNS can assist to lessen signs and symptoms of anxiety, melancholy, and exceptional mood troubles.

One of the main benefits of VNS for intellectual health is its capability to alter the frame's pressure response. When the vagus nerve is stimulated, it triggers the release of neurotransmitters like serotonin and dopamine, that would assist to lessen feelings of tension and despair. Additionally, VNS has been positioned to growth stages of GABA, a neurotransmitter that facilitates to calm the mind and reduce anxiety.

VNS has been studied as a remedy for a number of mental fitness conditions, which incorporates melancholy, tension, bipolar disease, and submit-annoying stress disease (PTSD). In scientific trials, VNS is robust in decreasing symptoms of despair and anxiety, and improving regular temper and extraordinary of lifestyles.

While VNS for intellectual health is still a considerably new situation of studies, the consequences to date are promising. As more studies is completed, VNS will probable grow to be an increasingly well-known and effective remedy desire for the ones struggling with highbrow fitness conditions.

Vagus Nerve Stimulation for Physical Health

Vagus nerve stimulation has additionally been demonstrated to have numerous benefits for bodily health. One of the maximum large blessings is its capability to reduce contamination in the body.

Studies have shown that VNS can reduce irritation through suppressing the manufacturing of cytokines, which may be proteins that promote contamination. This may also have a extremely good effect on a huge variety of fitness conditions, which include arthritis, bronchial allergic reactions, and inflammatory bowel disease.

VNS has furthermore been demonstrated to have a superb impact on heart fitness. It can help regulate coronary heart fee and blood stress, that could reduce the hazard of coronary heart disorder and stroke. VNS has been authorized with the resource of the FDA as a treatment for drug-resistant times of epilepsy and despair, and it's miles being studied as a capability remedy for coronary coronary heart failure.

Chapter 3: Disorders

The vagus nerve is answerable for regulating a fantastic sort of physical abilties, together with digestion, coronary coronary heart price, and breathing. When the vagus nerve is not functioning well, it is able to bring about quite a few health issues called vagus nerve problems.

Vagus nerve troubles may be because of severa factors, on the aspect of damage, sickness, or chronic pressure. Some of the maximum commonplace vagus nerve issues embody gastroparesis, that may be a condition that influences the stomach's capability to drain nicely, and vasovagal syncope, that could be a unexpected drop in blood stress that could cause fainting.

Other vagus nerve troubles include irritable bowel syndrome (IBS), that is a continual digestive ailment that could motive stomach ache, bloating, and constipation or diarrhea, and arrhythmia, this is an extraordinary heartbeat that might bring about dizziness, shortness of breath, and chest ache.

While vagus nerve troubles may be tough to live with, there are lots of treatment options to be had. These may additionally encompass medicines, way of lifestyles modifications, and self-care techniques which includes meditation, deep breathing sporting sports, and yoga.

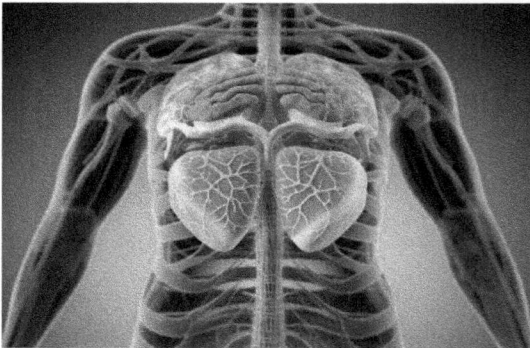

Common Vagus Nerve Disorders and Their Symptoms

When the vagus nerve is not functioning properly, it could purpose a whole lot of problems that might have a great impact on a person's notable of life.

One of the most common vagus nerve problems is gastroparesis, that is a state of affairs that affects the digestive device. Gastroparesis happens whilst the muscles inside the belly are unable to well settlement, that would reason quite various signs and symptoms and signs and symptoms consisting of nausea, vomiting, and belly pain.

Another not unusual vagus nerve ailment is vasovagal syncope, that's a state of affairs that motives fainting or loss of recognition. This disorder happens at the same time as the vagus nerve overreacts to nice triggers, including reputation up too brief or experiencing a surprising drop in blood pressure.

In addition to those issues, the vagus nerve moreover can be responsible for diverse different conditions together with epilepsy, despair, and anxiety. When the vagus nerve isn't functioning well, it is able to bring about some of signs which incorporates seizures, mood swings, and problem snoozing.

If you are experiencing any of those symptoms and signs and signs, it is vital to speak with a healthcare expert to decide if a vagus nerve disease is an underlying cause. With proper evaluation and remedy, many vagus nerve problems may be effectively controlled, permitting people to stay a whole and wholesome lifestyles.

Diagnosis and Treatment of Vagus Nerve Disorders

Diagnosing vagus nerve issues may be a hard assignment for healthcare specialists. This is because the signs of vagus nerve disorders may be vague and non-particular, making it difficult to pinpoint the best purpose of the problem. However, severa diagnostic tests may be finished to help grow to be privy to the underlying problem.

One of the most commonplace diagnostic tests for vagus nerve issues is an electrocardiogram (ECG). This test measures the electric interest of the coronary coronary heart and may help select out any abnormalities inside the coronary heart rhythm that can be because of vagus nerve sickness.

Another diagnostic check that may be used is an endoscopy. This entails putting a small digital digicam into the digestive tract to examine the esophagus, stomach, and small gut. This test can assist emerge as privy to any abnormalities within the digestive tract that can be as a result of vagus nerve dysfunction.

Once a evaluation has been made, remedy options for vagus nerve problems will rely on the underlying cause of the problem. In some instances, treatment may be prescribed to assist manipulate signs and symptoms and signs and symptoms together with nausea, vomiting, and heart palpitations.

In extra extreme instances, surgery can be vital to accurate the underlying hassle. For example, if a vagus nerve disease is as a consequence of a tumor or unique increase, surgery can be required to dispose of the growth and repair ordinary characteristic to the nerve.

In addition to scientific treatments, lifestyle changes, and self-care also may be effective in handling vagus nerve issues. This may additionally moreover consist of things like stress good buy techniques, dietary adjustments, and regular exercising.

Overall, on the equal time as vagus nerve problems may be hard to diagnose and address, there are loads of options to be had to help control signs and signs and signs and symptoms and signs and symptoms and decorate the brilliant of lifestyles for the ones dwelling with the ones conditions.

Lifestyle Changes and Self-Care for Vagus Nerve Disorders

When it includes managing vagus nerve troubles, lifestyle adjustments and self-care can play a important role in enhancing signs and commonplace best of existence. Here are some suggestions and techniques to take into account:

1. Practice Deep Breathing: Deep respiratory sports activities can assist stimulate the vagus nerve and sell relaxation. Try inhaling deeply via your nose for a rely of four, retaining for a rely of 4, and exhaling slowly thru your mouth for a rely of six. Repeat this for numerous minutes each day.

2. Get Regular Exercise: Exercise has been shown to beautify vagal tone, it is the diploma of the way well the vagus nerve is functioning. Aim for at the least thirty mins of mild exercise maximum days of the week.

three. Reduce Stress: Chronic strain can negatively impact the vagus nerve and exacerbate signs and symptoms and signs and symptoms and signs and symptoms of vagus nerve issues. Consider incorporating stress-lowering sports into your every day routine, which includes yoga, meditation, or spending time in nature.

4. Improve Digestive Health: The vagus nerve plays a key role in digestive characteristic, so it is vital to guide your gut health. This can include ingesting a balanced diet with masses of fiber, staying hydrated, and warding off cause meals that could exacerbate signs.

5. Prioritize Sleep: Getting enough restful sleep is critical for traditional health and also can help improve vagus nerve characteristic. Aim for seven to 9 hours of sleep every night and installation a regular bedtime everyday.

By making the ones way of lifestyles modifications and running in the direction of self-care, you can help assist your vagus nerve and control signs of vagus nerve troubles.

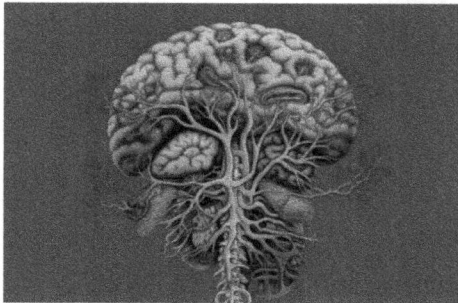

6. Vagus Nerve and the Gut-Brain Axis

Understanding the Gut-Brain Axis

The intestine-mind axis is a complex communique community that connects the treasured concerned device (CNS) with the enteric apprehensive device (ENS), this is liable for regulating the digestive device. The intestine-mind axis consists of bidirectional communique a few of the mind and the gut, with alerts visiting in both commands.

The gut-mind axis performs a important position in maintaining ordinary fitness and well-being. It is liable for regulating digestion, nutrient absorption, and immune characteristic, in addition to influencing temper and behavior. The intestine is frequently referred to as the "second thoughts" as it contains tens of tens of tens of millions of neurons that communicate with the brain through the vagus nerve.

The intestine-mind axis is likewise endorsed with the aid of the gut microbiome, that's a complicated network of microorganisms that inhabit the digestive tract. The intestine microbiome performs a critical role in regulating immune characteristic, digestion, and metabolism, and has been associated with a whole lot of health situations, together with weight problems, diabetes, and inflammatory bowel illness.

Understanding the gut-thoughts axis is important for keeping optimum fitness and properly-being. By promoting a wholesome gut microbiome and supporting vagus nerve characteristic, we're able to beautify digestion, enhance immune feature, and reduce the danger of an entire lot of health conditions.

The Role of the Vagus Nerve inside the Gut-Brain Axis

The vagus nerve is the primary pathway for communication many of the gut and the thoughts.

It is chargeable for regulating various physical features, together with heart fee, respiration, and digestion. When it involves the gut-brain axis, the vagus nerve acts as a -manner verbal exchange pathway, sending indicators from the gut to the thoughts and vice versa.

One of the primary features of the vagus nerve in the intestine-thoughts axis is to alter digestion. It does this with the aid of the use of way of controlling the release of digestive enzymes and regulating the motion of meals through the digestive tract. Additionally, the vagus nerve plays a feature inside the gut's immune response, supporting to protect in the direction of risky pathogens.

Beyond its position in digestion and immunity, the vagus nerve furthermore performs a essential function in regulating temper and emotions. It is chargeable for the discharge of neurotransmitters like serotonin and dopamine, which can be important for regulating temper and feelings. Studies have demonstrated that stimulating the vagus nerve can have a pleasing impact on intellectual health, reducing signs and signs and symptoms of hysteria and depression.

Vagus Nerve Stimulation and its Effects on the Gut-Brain Axis

Vagus nerve stimulation (VNS) is a manner that involves the use of electric impulses to stimulate the vagus nerve. This approach has been used for decades to address severa scientific situations, collectively with epilepsy, depression, and migraines. However, contemporary studies has confirmed that VNS can also have a notable impact at the gut-mind axis.

Studies have verified that VNS can decorate intestine motility, reduce infection, and growth the production of useful gut micro organism. This is due to the reality the vagus nerve performs a crucial role in regulating the digestive device. When the vagus nerve is stimulated, it sends signs to the thoughts, which in turn turns on the parasympathetic apprehensive device. This tool is accountable for promoting relaxation, which is important for proper digestion.

In addition to its results at the digestive device, VNS has also been proven to have a outstanding effect on intellectual health. Research has proven that VNS can lessen signs and symptoms and signs and symptoms of hysteria and melancholy, which are regularly related to gut health. This is because of the truth the gut and thoughts are carefully related, and changes in you can have an effect on the other.

The Connection many of the Vagus Nerve and Digestive Disorders

The vagus nerve plays a important function in the digestive device, connecting the thoughts to the gut and regulating numerous digestive abilties. When the vagus nerve is functioning nicely, it permits to sell healthful digestion and prevent digestive issues. However, at the identical time because the vagus nerve is broken or not functioning properly, it can cause a whole lot of digestive troubles.

One of the most not unusual digestive troubles related to the vagus nerve is gastroparesis, a scenario in which the stomach isn't capable of empty nicely. This can reason signs and symptoms and symptoms and signs and symptoms which includes nausea, vomiting, bloating, and stomach ache. Studies have installed that vagus nerve harm or sickness is a common reason of gastroparesis.

In addition to gastroparesis, the vagus nerve is also concerned in other digestive issues together with irritable bowel syndrome (IBS), inflammatory bowel sickness (IBD), and gastroesophageal reflux illness (GERD). In IBS, the vagus nerve can be overactive or underactive, main to signs together with belly ache, bloating, and diarrhea or constipation. In IBD, the vagus nerve may additionally play a position in regulating inflammation within the intestine, and vagus nerve stimulation has been established to have anti inflammatory results.

GERD, as a substitute, is a situation in which belly acid flows all over again into the esophagus, causing heartburn and different signs and signs and signs. The vagus nerve lets in to adjust the characteristic of the decrease esophageal sphincter, it is chargeable for stopping stomach acid from flowing again into the esophagus. When the vagus nerve isn't always functioning properly, this could purpose GERD.

Overall, the relationship between the vagus nerve and digestive troubles is complicated and multifaceted. While extra research is wanted to fully apprehend the placement of the vagus nerve in digestive health, it's miles clean that keeping healthy vagus nerve function is important for preventing and handling digestive issues.

The Vagus Nerve and Mental Health: Anxiety and Depression

The relationship among the vagus nerve and intellectual health is a topic of growing interest among researchers and healthcare specialists. The vagus nerve plays a important role in regulating the frame's pressure response and emotional nation, making it a capability goal for treating tension and melancholy.

Studies have confirmed that people with anxiety and melancholy frequently have impaired vagal tone, which refers back to the electricity and responsiveness of the vagus nerve. This can motive numerous symptoms and signs, which include expanded coronary coronary heart price, shallow respiration, and digestive troubles.

Vagus nerve stimulation (VNS) has emerged as a promising remedy for anxiety and melancholy. VNS consists of the use of a small device this is implanted inside the frame and elements electric impulses to the vagus nerve. This can assist to alter the body's strain reaction and enhance mood.

Chapter 4: Heart Health

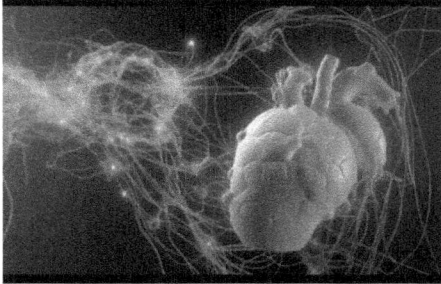

Understanding the Role of the Vagus Nerve in Heart Health

The vagus nerve is chargeable for regulating the body's "rest and digest" reaction. This nerve plays a massive position in coronary heart health with the aid of way of controlling the coronary heart charge, blood strain, and coronary heart fee variability.

The vagus nerve slows the coronary coronary heart fee and reduces blood strain, it's crucial for preserving a healthful heart. When the vagus nerve is activated, it releases acetylcholine, which permits to loosen up the blood vessels and decrease infection within the body.

Research has tested that humans with a higher coronary heart charge variability (HRV) have a decrease hazard of growing coronary coronary heart sickness. HRV refers to the version in time among every heartbeat, and it is an indicator of the body's potential to adapt to strain. The vagus nerve plays a essential feature in regulating HRV, and stimulating this nerve can beautify HRV and decrease the chance of coronary coronary heart disease.

Furthermore, the vagus nerve is involved within the law of the immune device, which can effect coronary coronary heart fitness. Chronic contamination inside the body can purpose the improvement of atherosclerosis, that is a circumstance wherein plaque builds up within the arteries and might bring about coronary heart attacks and strokes. By lowering infection within the body, the vagus nerve can help to prevent the development of atherosclerosis and remarkable coronary coronary coronary heart situations.

The Connection Between Vagus Nerve Stimulation and Heart Rate Variability

The connection among vagus nerve stimulation and heart rate variability is an important element of knowledge the feature of the vagus nerve in coronary coronary heart health. Heart price variability refers to the model in time amongst each heartbeat, and it's far an critical indicator of ordinary coronary coronary heart fitness.

When the vagus nerve is inspired, it sends indicators to the coronary heart to sluggish down and reduce heart charge. This consequences in advanced coronary heart fee variability, it is related to better coronary coronary heart health outcomes.

Research has established that vagus nerve stimulation can be an powerful treatment for coronary coronary heart situations together with atrial traumatic inflammation and coronary heart failure. By stimulating the vagus nerve, the coronary coronary heart rate may be regulated and stepped forward, important to better preferred coronary heart fitness.

Furthermore, vagus nerve stimulation has been confirmed to have advantages past surely coronary heart fee variability. It also can reduce contamination, decorate blood strain, and reduce stress ranges, all of which might be essential elements in preserving a healthy coronary heart.

Vagus Nerve Stimulation as a Treatment for Heart Conditions

Vagus nerve stimulation is a promising remedy for numerous coronary coronary heart conditions. This is due to the fact the vagus nerve performs a crucial function in regulating the heart's rhythm and function. When the vagus nerve is inspired, it is able to sluggish down the coronary coronary coronary heart fee and reduce the workload on the coronary coronary coronary heart.

One of the most commonplace coronary coronary heart conditions that vagus nerve stimulation is used to deal with is atrial disturbing inflammation. Atrial fibrillation is a situation in which the coronary coronary heart beats irregularly and can motive blood clots, stroke, and coronary heart failure. Vagus nerve stimulation is powerful in lowering the frequency and severity of atrial worrying infection episodes.

Vagus nerve stimulation has moreover been used to address coronary coronary heart failure. Heart failure is a circumstance wherein the coronary coronary heart isn't capable of pump blood effectively, important to fatigue, shortness of breath, and different signs and signs. Vagus nerve stimulation can help improve coronary heart feature by means of manner of using reducing infection and oxidative stress, that would damage the coronary coronary heart muscle.

In addition to the ones situations, vagus nerve stimulation has additionally been studied as a functionality remedy for immoderate blood pressure, angina, and one-of-a-kind cardiovascular sicknesses. While more research is needed to simply apprehend the blessings of vagus nerve stimulation for coronary heart health, the results up to now are promising.

The Benefits of Vagus Nerve Stimulation for Heart Health

Vagus nerve stimulation has been proven to have severa blessings for coronary coronary heart health. One of the most considerable benefits is its functionality to lessen irritation inside the frame. Inflammation is a first-rate contributor to coronary coronary coronary heart illness, and through lowering infection, vagus nerve stimulation can help save you the improvement of coronary heart sickness.

Another benefit of vagus nerve stimulation is its capability to regulate heart charge and blood stress. By stimulating the vagus nerve, the body can maintain a healthful stability the numerous sympathetic and parasympathetic worried systems, which can be liable for regulating coronary heart fee and blood strain. This can assist prevent conditions which incorporates hypertension and arrhythmia.

In addition to the ones advantages, vagus nerve stimulation has additionally been shown to beautify trendy coronary heart feature. This is because of its ability to boom blood go along with the glide to the coronary coronary coronary heart and enhance the heart's capability to pump blood successfully.

Techniques for Stimulating the Vagus Nerve to Improve Heart Health

Several strategies may be used to stimulate the vagus nerve and enhance coronary coronary heart health. One of the best approaches is thru deep respiratory physical video games. Slow, deep breaths can spark off the vagus nerve and help to regulate coronary coronary heart charge and blood strain. It's important to cognizance on breathing from the diaphragm, in desire to shallow chest respiratory.

Another method is meditation and mindfulness practices. These practices were demonstrated to increase vagal tone, that is the electricity of the vagus nerve's reaction to stimulation. This can result in improved coronary coronary heart charge variability and everyday coronary heart health.

Acupuncture is each other method that may be used to stimulate the vagus nerve. This historic exercise consists of the insertion of thin needles into particular elements at the body. These elements correspond to splendid organs and systems within the body, which encompass the coronary heart and the vagus nerve.

Finally, there are gadgets available that can be used to stimulate the vagus nerve. These gadgets are generally implanted below the pores and skin and use electric impulses to set off the nerve. They are effective in treating positive coronary coronary heart conditions, inclusive of coronary coronary heart failure and arrhythmias.

Future Directions in Vagus Nerve Research for Heart Health

As research on the vagus nerve and its position in heart fitness maintains to comply, there are numerous exciting recommendations that scientists are exploring. One area of interest is the use of non-invasive techniques to stimulate the vagus nerve. While present day-day strategies include invasive strategies which embody surgical treatment or implantation of a tool, researchers are investigating methods to stimulate the nerve the usage of outside devices or perhaps sound waves.

Another promising road of research is using vagus nerve stimulation in aggregate with different recovery techniques. For instance, studies have established that combining vagus nerve stimulation with traditional drug recovery methods can bring about advanced consequences for sufferers with coronary

coronary heart situations together with coronary coronary coronary heart failure.

Additionally, researchers are exploring the capability of the vagus nerve as a target for present day drug treatments. By growing tablets that especially goal the vagus nerve, scientists wish to create greater effective remedies for coronary heart situations which might be currently tough to govern.

Overall, the destiny of vagus nerve research for coronary coronary heart health is vibrant. As scientists keep to discover the numerous approaches wherein the vagus nerve affects coronary heart feature, we can assume to look new and modern treatments emerge so one can help enhance the lives of tens of lots and thousands of human beings spherical the arena.

Chapter 5: Respiratory System

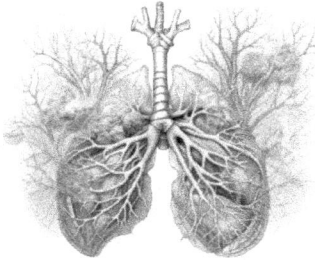

The Vagus Nerve and Respiratory System

One of the important factor areas that the vagus nerve impacts is the respiratory gadget. The breathing tool is accountable for the change of oxygen and carbon dioxide inside the body. It includes the lungs, airways, and muscle tissues that manage respiratory. The vagus nerve performs a essential role in regulating the respiratory device thru controlling the fee and depth of respiratory, in addition to the rest and contraction of the airways.

When the vagus nerve is stimulated, it could cause the airways to dilate, bearing in mind a good deal less complex respiration. It can also sluggish down the respiratory price and increase the depth of each breath. This is crucial in conditions wherein the frame needs to conserve electricity, together with within the direction of sleep or instances of rest.

On the opportunity hand, whilst the vagus nerve is inhibited, it could cause the airlines to constrict, making it more tough to breathe. This can show up for the duration of times of stress or anxiety even as the body is in a fight-or-flight mode.

Understanding the relationship a few of the vagus nerve and the respiratory system is vital for treating respiratory problems which include allergies, persistent obstructive pulmonary sickness (COPD), and sleep apnea. By concentrated on the vagus nerve via severa remedies, which incorporates vagus nerve stimulation, it's far feasible to decorate respiration function and first-class of lifestyles for human beings with those situations.

In this monetary disaster, we can find out the anatomy and frame shape of the vagus nerve and respiratory device, in addition to the location of the vagus nerve in respiratory control. We may also even look at the scientific packages of vagus nerve stimulation in respiratory treatment and the future of this exciting place.

Anatomy and Physiology of the Vagus Nerve and Respiratory System

The vagus nerve is a key player within the autonomic concerned device, which controls a number of the frame's computerized functions, collectively with respiratory. The breathing machine, however, is answerable for the alternate of oxygen and carbon dioxide within the body.

The vagus nerve has branches which may be involved in breathing control: the advanced laryngeal nerve and the recurrent laryngeal nerve. The superior laryngeal nerve innervates the muscles that manage the hollow and closing of the vocal cords, at the same time because the recurrent laryngeal nerve innervates the muscle companies that control the motion of the vocal cords for the duration of respiration.

The breathing machine is made from the lungs, airlines, and muscular tissues involved in respiratory. The lungs are the primary organs answerable for fuel change, at the same time as the airways (together with the trachea, bronchi, and bronchioles) delivery air to and from the lungs. The muscle companies worried in breathing encompass the diaphragm and intercostal muscle companies, which work together to increase and agreement the chest hole area.

The vagus nerve performs an active position in coordinating the activity of those respiration muscle companies. When we inhale, the diaphragm contracts, and the intercostal muscle tissues enlarge the chest hole location, permitting air to circulate the lungs. When we exhale, the diaphragm and intercostal muscle agencies relax, allowing air to float out of the lungs. The vagus nerve enables to modify the timing and intensity of these muscle contractions, ensuring that we breathe efficiently and efficiently.

Overall, the anatomy and frame structure of the vagus nerve and respiratory system are carefully intertwined. The vagus nerve performs a essential function in respiratory control, coordinating the hobby of the muscle tissues worried in breathing and ensuring that we get the oxygen we need to stay to tell the tale.

The Role of the Vagus Nerve in Respiratory Control

The vagus nerve is responsible for regulating the price and depth of respiratory, further to the change of gases within the lungs. The vagus nerve is a number one trouble of the parasympathetic apprehensive tool, this is accountable for the frame's rest and digest response.

When we inhale, the vagus nerve sends indicators to the brainstem, which then turns on the respiration muscle tissues to enlarge the lungs and fill them with air. Similarly, while we exhale, the vagus nerve indicators the brainstem to loosen up the respiratory muscle tissues and expel the air from the lungs. This method is known as respiration rhythmogenesis and is crucial for keeping proper oxygen and carbon dioxide degrees in the frame.

The vagus nerve furthermore plays a function in regulating the diameter of the airways within the lungs. It does this thru controlling the easy muscle that surrounds the airlines, which could constrict or dilate relying on the frame's goals. This is important in conditions which encompass bronchial allergies, wherein the airlines can end up inflamed and narrowed, making it hard to breathe. Vagus nerve stimulation is strong in reducing airway constriction and enhancing breathing in people with allergic reactions.

In addition to its characteristic in breathing manipulate, the vagus nerve furthermore plays a function in the body's reaction to pressure. When we're below pressure, the sympathetic tense gadget is activated, that might growth coronary heart fee and blood pressure. The vagus nerve acts as a counterbalance to this reaction via activating the parasympathetic demanding device, which slows the coronary coronary coronary heart charge and promotes rest. This is called the vagal brake and is an critical mechanism for keeping homeostasis within the body.

Vagus Nerve Stimulation and Respiratory Disorders

Vagus nerve stimulation (VNS) has been shown to have a significant impact on breathing troubles.

One of the maximum commonplace breathing issues that may be handled with VNS is obstructive sleep apnea (OSA). OSA is a scenario wherein the airway turns into blocked in the route of sleep, causing the individual to stop respiratory for brief durations of time. VNS can assist to reduce the severity of OSA through developing muscle tone within the airway and improving respiration styles.

VNS has additionally been tested to be effective in treating chronic obstructive pulmonary disorder (COPD). COPD is a modern-day lung illness that makes it hard to breathe. VNS can assist to enhance lung characteristic and reduce the severity of signs together with shortness of breath and coughing.

In addition to OSA and COPD, VNS has been used to address distinct respiratory troubles which include hypersensitive reactions and bronchitis. By stimulating the vagus nerve, VNS can assist to reduce contamination inside the airways and decorate respiratory function.

Overall, VNS has proven exceptional promise inside the treatment of respiratory issues. As extra research is executed, VNS will probable become an increasingly critical device in breathing remedy.

Clinical Applications of Vagus Nerve Stimulation in Respiratory Therapy

Clinical applications of vagus nerve stimulation in respiration remedy have tested promising outcomes inside the remedy of numerous respiratory issues. One such infection is chronic obstructive pulmonary disease (COPD), that is characterised with the useful resource of persistent obstruction of airflow inside the lungs. Studies have shown that vagus nerve stimulation can enhance lung function and reduce the frequency of exacerbations in sufferers with COPD.

Another respiration ailment that may advantage from vagus nerve stimulation is bronchial asthma. Asthma is a persistent inflammatory sickness of the airways that would purpose wheezing, shortness of breath, and chest tightness. Vagus nerve stimulation has been tested to lessen airway infection and beautify lung characteristic in patients with bronchial allergic reactions.

Vagus nerve stimulation has additionally been studied as a capability treatment for sleep apnea, a ailment characterized with the aid of pauses in respiratory at some stage in sleep. Studies have proven that vagus nerve stimulation can enhance sleep splendid and reduce the severity of sleep apnea in patients.

9. Vagus Nerve and Immune System

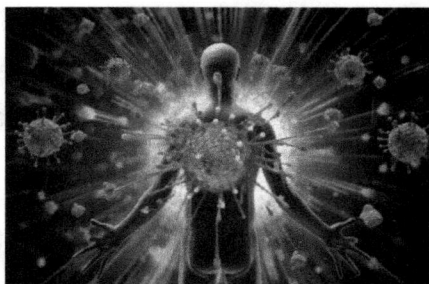

Understanding the Role of the Vagus Nerve in Immune Function

The immune machine is a complex network of cells, tissues, and organs that art work collectively to guard the frame from unstable pathogens and overseas invaders. It is liable for identifying and disposing of threats to our health, in conjunction with viruses, micro organism, and most cancers cells. However, the immune device can also become overactive and assault wholesome cells and tissues, vital to autoimmune diseases.

The vagus nerve enables to control contamination, it virtually is a crucial approach within the immune reaction. Inflammation is the frame's natural reaction to damage or contamination, but even as it will become continual, it could bring about pretty a variety of fitness problems, consisting of autoimmune illnesses, hypersensitive reactions, or even depression.

Research has established that the vagus nerve can help to alter infection via releasing neurotransmitters that hose down the immune reaction. This approach is called the cholinergic anti inflammatory pathway. By activating this pathway, the vagus nerve can help to reduce contamination and sell recuperation.

In addition to its feature in infection, the vagus nerve is also concerned inside the intestine-mind axis, this is the relationship many of the digestive system and the main concerned device. The intestine is domestic to trillions of bacteria, which play a important function in immune function. The vagus nerve enables to alter the stableness of those bacteria, which could have a big effect on immune health.

Overall, the vagus nerve is a key issue of the immune tool, and understanding its position in immune function is essential for maintaining maximum appropriate health. In the following sections, we are capable of explore the connection a number of the vagus nerve and infection, the gut-mind axis, and the functionality healing applications of vagus nerve stimulation for immune-related problems.

The Vagus Nerve and Inflammation: How It Affects the Immune System

When the immune system detects a threat, consisting of an endemic or micro organism, it triggers an inflammatory reaction to assist fight off the invader. However, if infection will become chronic or immoderate, it can motive pretty a number health problems, in conjunction with autoimmune troubles, allergic reactions, or maybe most cancers.

The vagus nerve allows to modulate this inflammatory reaction with the resource of way of sending signs and symptoms to the thoughts that assist to modify the hobby of immune cells. Specifically, the vagus nerve stimulates the discharge of neurotransmitters, together with acetylcholine, that could inhibit the manufacturing of pro-inflammatory cytokines, which might be molecules that promote infection.

In addition, the vagus nerve can also stimulate the producing of anti-inflammatory cytokines, which help to dampen the immune reaction and sell recovery. This stability amongst pro-inflammatory and anti-inflammatory signs is essential for preserving maximum brilliant immune function and stopping chronic contamination.

Research has proven that disorder of the vagus nerve can make a contribution to some of immune-related disorders, which incorporates inflammatory bowel disease, rheumatoid arthritis, and sepsis. By data the region of the vagus nerve in contamination and immune feature, we can enlarge new remedies that focus on this pathway to assist deal with the ones situations.

The Gut-Brain Axis: The Connection Between the Vagus Nerve and Immune Health

The intestine-thoughts axis is a complex verbal exchange network that links the essential worried tool to the gastrointestinal tract. This connection is facilitated through the vagus nerve, which plays a critical position in regulating immune characteristic. The intestine is home to trillions of microorganisms, together referred to as the intestine microbiota, which play a critical characteristic in retaining the health of the immune machine.

The intestine microbiota communicates with the immune device thru the gut-mind axis, this is regulated via the use of the vagus nerve. The vagus nerve acts as a -manner street, transmitting alerts from the intestine to the brain and vice versa. This verbal exchange community permits the immune device to reply to changes in the intestine microbiota and preserve a healthy stability of immune cells.

Research has proven that gut microbiota will have an effect at the development and function of immune cells, which incorporates T cells, B cells, and natural killer cells. These immune cells play a crucial role in protecting the body in opposition to pathogens and retaining immune homeostasis. Dysregulation of the intestine microbiota can cause immune ailment and boom the chance of autoimmune illnesses, hypersensitive reactions, and other immune-related issues.

The vagus nerve additionally performs a position in regulating the gut microbiota. Studies have shown that vagus nerve stimulation can adjust the composition of the intestine microbiota, main to a reduction in infection and advanced immune feature. This shows that the intestine-thoughts axis and the vagus nerve may be potential desires for the development of new treatment options for immune-related problems.

Vagus Nerve Stimulation: A Promising Therapy for Immune-Related Disorders

VNS has been explored as a capacity remedy for immune-associated problems.

Research has shown that VNS can modulate the immune device via way of manner of lowering infection and growing the manufacturing of anti-inflammatory cytokines. This is completed through the activation of the cholinergic anti inflammatory pathway, this is mediated via manner of the vagus nerve.

In a have a examine posted within the mag Bioelectronic Medicine, researchers placed that VNS grow to be effective in decreasing irritation in patients with rheumatoid arthritis. The have a look at concerned using a small device that modified into implanted in the affected person's neck to stimulate the vagus nerve. After six months of treatment, the patients confirmed massive upgrades in their symptoms, which consist of reduced joint ache and swelling.

Another have a have a take a look at posted within the journal Brain, Behavior, and Immunity positioned that VNS grow to be effective in reducing infection in patients with Crohn's ailment. The examine worried using a non-invasive VNS device that grow to be positioned on the affected person's ear. After 4 weeks of remedy, the sufferers showed first rate improvements of their symptoms and signs, which incorporates reduced infection and superior high-quality of life.

While VNS remains considered an experimental remedy for immune-related issues, the results of those research are promising. Further research is needed to determine the ideal parameters for VNS remedy and to pick out which patients are most probable to gain from this treatment. Nonetheless, VNS represents a promising new approach to treating immune-related issues and can provide need to patients who've no longer responded to conventional treatments.

Lifestyle Factors That Affect Vagus Nerve Function and Immune Health

Lifestyle elements play a great characteristic inside the health of our immune device and the feature of our vagus nerve. Here are some key way of life elements that could have an impact on vagus nerve characteristic and immune health.

Chapter 6: Mental Health

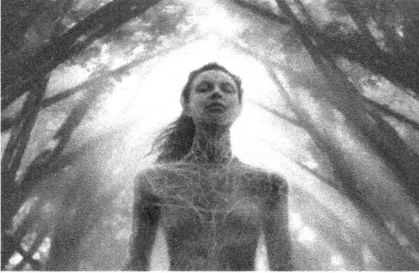

Understanding the Role of the Vagus Nerve in Mental Health

In modern years, researchers have decided that the vagus nerve furthermore plays a huge position in our intellectual fitness. The nerve is answerable for regulating our pressure reaction and assisting us to revel in calm and relaxed. When the vagus nerve is functioning well, it may assist us to control pressure and tension, decorate our temper, and even enhance our cognitive competencies.

However, whilst the vagus nerve isn't functioning properly, it may result in pretty

pretty quite a number intellectual health problems, which incorporates depression, tension, and post-demanding pressure illness (PTSD). This is because of the truth the nerve is carefully linked to our frame's strain response device, which could become overactive and cause persistent stress and inflammation.

Understanding the characteristic of the vagus nerve in mental fitness is critical for all of us attempting to find to beautify their regular nicely-being. By mastering the way to stimulate the nerve and guide its proper functioning, we're capable of take steps to lessen strain, enhance our temper, and decorate our highbrow readability.

The Vagus Nerve and the Stress Response: How it Impacts Mental Health

The vagus nerve plays a critical function in regulating the frame's strain response. When we experience strain, the sympathetic stressful device is activated, triggering the "fight or flight" response. However, the vagus nerve acts as a counterbalance to this response, selling rest and lowering the physiological effects of stress.

Research has hooked up that people with low vagal tone, or decreased interest of the vagus nerve, are more at risk of strain-related intellectual fitness problems together with tension and depression. This is because the vagus nerve is responsible for regulating the release of pressure hormones at the side of cortisol and adrenaline, and moreover allows to lessen contamination inside the frame.

When the vagus nerve is functioning optimally, it can help to reduce the signs and signs and symptoms and signs and symptoms of pressure-associated intellectual health problems. This is why strategies which incorporates deep respiratory, meditation, and yoga, which stimulate the vagus nerve, are effective in decreasing tension and despair.

On the other hand, continual strain can bring about a dysregulation of the vagus nerve, ensuing in a discounted capability to deal with strain and an improved chance of growing intellectual fitness issues. This is why it's miles essential to prioritize stress management techniques that sell vagal tone, consisting of ordinary workout, social help, and mindfulness practices.

The Gut-Brain Connection: The Vagus Nerve's Role in Digestion and Mental Health

The gut-mind connection is a captivating vicinity of study that has obtained lots of interest in modern-day years. The vagus nerve performs a important role in this connection, as it's miles responsible for transmitting records some of the gut and the thoughts.

The gut is regularly called the "2nd thoughts" because it includes tens of loads of thousands of neurons that communicate with the mind through the vagus nerve. This verbal exchange is bidirectional, that means that the thoughts can effect the gut, and the gut can have an impact at the mind.

Research has verified that the health of our intestine is intently associated with our highbrow health. For example, individuals with irritable bowel syndrome (IBS) often enjoy symptoms inclusive of tension and melancholy. This is because of the truth the intestine and the mind percent some of the same neurotransmitters, together with serotonin and dopamine.

When the gut isn't always functioning properly, it can result in an imbalance of those neurotransmitters, which could damage our highbrow fitness. This is in which the vagus nerve is available in.

The vagus nerve permits to adjust digestion thru controlling the release of digestive enzymes and the movement of food via the digestive tract. It moreover plays a feature inside the intestine's immune reaction and lets in to maintain the integrity of the gut lining.

When the vagus nerve is stimulated, it could have a excessive quality effect on our intellectual fitness. This is because the stimulation of the nerve triggers the release of neurotransmitters together with acetylcholine, which has been tested to have an anti-inflammatory impact at the frame.

In addition to vagus nerve stimulation, there are specific methods to enhance the health of our intestine and, in turn, our highbrow fitness. These embody eating a healthy weight loss program, getting sufficient sleep, and reducing pressure levels.

By understanding the position of the vagus nerve inside the gut-thoughts connection, we will take steps to enhance our highbrow fitness by using the usage of improving the health of our gut. This is an interesting location of research that has the capability to revolutionize the manner we don't forget intellectual health and its connection to the relaxation of the body.

Vagus Nerve Stimulation: A Promising Treatment for Mental Health Disorders

The vagus nerve is responsible for controlling the parasympathetic nervous gadget, which allows to calm the frame and mind sooner or later of times of strain. When the vagus nerve is not functioning well, it could bring about more than a few highbrow fitness troubles along with tension, melancholy, and placed up-disturbing pressure contamination (PTSD).

Fortunately, there is a promising remedy that has emerged in present day years that entails stimulating the vagus nerve. This remedy is known as vagus nerve stimulation (VNS) and consists of the use of a small device this is implanted in the body to deliver electric powered powered impulses to the vagus nerve.

Research has proven that VNS can be effective in treating some of highbrow health disorders. For instance, studies have decided that VNS can substantially reduce signs and symptoms and signs and symptoms and symptoms of depression in patients who have not answered to traditional treatments which incorporates treatment and remedy. VNS has moreover been determined to be powerful in treating anxiety troubles, PTSD, or maybe schizophrenia.

One of the crucial element advantages of VNS is that it's far a non-invasive remedy that doesn't comprise remedy. This makes it an attractive desire for patients who may be hesitant to take remedy due to problems about issue consequences or dependancy.

Mind-Body Practices to Stimulate the Vagus Nerve and Improve Mental Health

Various thoughts-frame practices can assist stimulate the vagus nerve and decorate intellectual fitness. These practices may be without problems covered into one's day by day habitual and might have a top notch impact on reducing pressure and tension levels.

One such workout is deep breathing sports activities sports. Deep respiratory includes taking slow, deep breaths from the diaphragm, in area of shallow breaths from the chest. This form of respiration activates the vagus nerve and triggers the relaxation response in the frame. Practicing deep respiratory for only some minutes an afternoon can help lessen stress and tension levels.

Another exercise that could stimulate the vagus nerve is yoga. Yoga involves a combination of bodily postures, breathing carrying sports, and meditation. The bodily postures and respiratory bodily sports assist activate the vagus nerve, at the equal time because the meditation issue permits calm the mind and reduce strain degrees. Practicing yoga regularly has been tested to decorate intellectual health and reduce symptoms of tension and depression.

Meditation and mindfulness practices also can assist stimulate the vagus nerve and decorate intellectual health. These practices involve that specialize in the prevailing 2nd and cultivating a revel in of reputation and elegance. By schooling mindfulness, people can discover ways to regulate their feelings and reduce pressure ranges, that might have a top notch impact on highbrow health.

Finally, accomplishing sports activities that promote social connection and powerful emotions can also stimulate the vagus nerve and enhance intellectual fitness. Activities which consist of spending time with cherished ones, volunteering, and training gratitude can all assist set off the vagus nerve and promote emotions of well-being and happiness.

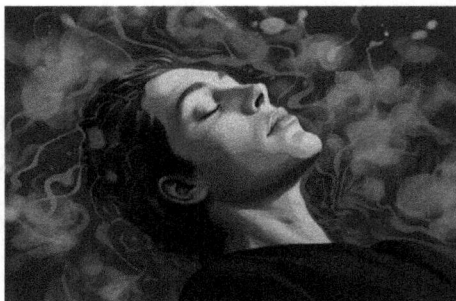

Epilepsy

The vagus nerve may have a large effect on neurological situations collectively with epilepsy.

Epilepsy is a neurological illness characterized by using using the use of recurrent seizures, that may variety from moderate to excessive and can have an impact on human beings of each age. While the proper causes of epilepsy are not without a doubt understood, it's far concept to be associated with bizarre electric pastime within the mind.

The vagus nerve has been observed to have a considerable effect on epilepsy, with studies showing that stimulation of the nerve can help reduce the frequency and severity of seizures. This has precipitated the improvement of vagus nerve stimulation remedy, a treatment that involves implanting a device that gives electric powered impulses to the nerve.

While vagus nerve stimulation therapy has shown promise in treating epilepsy, it isn't with out dangers and capacity factor consequences. As such, opportunity remedy plans that concentrate on the vagus nerve, at the side of meditation and breathing physical sports, also are being explored.

As research into the vagus nerve and its role in epilepsy maintains, it is was hoping that new remedies and remedies may be advanced that could help enhance the lives of those dwelling with this circumstance.

Understanding the Role of the Vagus Nerve in Epilepsy

Recent studies has shown that the vagus nerve is concerned in the improvement and manage of epilepsy.

Chapter 7: Alternative Therapies For Epilepsy

While vagus nerve stimulation remedy has set up promise in treating epilepsy, it is not the only possibility to be had. There are opportunity treatment plans that target the vagus nerve and can provide remedy for those with epilepsy.

One such treatment is transcutaneous vagus nerve stimulation (TVNS). This includes using a small electric tool that is located at the skin over the vagus nerve. The tool sends electric powered impulses to the nerve, which could assist reduce seizures in some people with epilepsy.

Another opportunity therapy is auricular vagus nerve stimulation (AVNS). This includes using a small device that is positioned at the ear and stimulates the vagus nerve thru the auricular branch. Like TVNS, AVNS has proven promise in reducing seizures in a few humans with epilepsy.

In addition to the ones non-invasive treatment alternatives, there also are surgical alternatives for concentrated on the vagus nerve. One such choice is vagus nerve resection, which includes the removal of a portion of the nerve. This manner is typically reserved for people with extreme epilepsy who've not spoke back to different treatments.

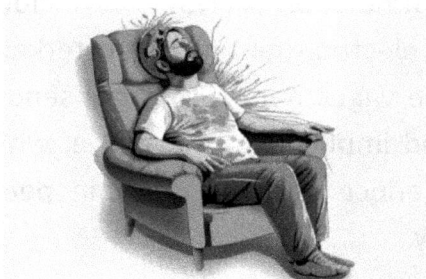

It is important to check that at the identical time as those possibility remedies may be powerful for some humans with epilepsy, they're now not a remedy. It is essential to artwork closely with a healthcare company to decide the tremendous treatment plan for each man or woman's unique desires. As research into the vagus nerve and its position in epilepsy continues, new recuperation techniques may additionally moreover moreover emerge that could offer even greater alternatives for those residing with this example.

Stroke

In state-of-the-art years, researchers have found that the vagus nerve additionally has a full-size impact on stroke restoration.

A stroke is a scientific emergency that takes area even as blood float to the brain is interrupted, either because of a blood clot or a ruptured blood vessel. This interruption can reason mind cells to die, essential to everlasting mind damage or perhaps loss of life. Strokes are a prime cause of disability and demise worldwide, affecting masses of lots of humans every one year.

The vagus nerve is involved in the frame's response to stroke. When the thoughts is damaged thru a stroke, the vagus nerve sends signals to the immune device, triggering an inflammatory response. This reaction can each help or harm the thoughts, relying at the severity and duration of the infection.

Researchers have determined that stimulating the vagus nerve can help lessen infection and sell stroke healing. Vagus nerve stimulation consists of sending electric powered impulses to the nerve, that could help modify the immune reaction and sell the growth of new thoughts cells.

In this bankruptcy, we can find out the function of the vagus nerve in stroke, the relationship among vagus nerve stimulation and stroke healing, and the capability risks and trouble outcomes of this remedy. We will also have a examine the extraordinarily-cutting-edge-day medical trials and studies on vagus nerve stimulation for stroke and communicate the future of this promising treatment preference.

Understanding the Role of the Vagus Nerve in Relation to Strokes

According to researchers, the vagus nerve plays a vast feature in stroke healing.

During a stroke, blood glide to the mind is disrupted, main to thoughts damage and functionality prolonged-term incapacity. The vagus nerve is involved inside the frame's response to this damage, particularly in the inflammatory reaction. Inflammation is a herbal reaction to harm, but inside the case of a stroke, it may cause further damage to the brain tissue.

The vagus nerve can assist modify this inflammatory reaction with the useful aid of releasing anti inflammatory entrepreneurs, that can assist reduce the damage due to stroke. Additionally, the vagus nerve can also assist modify blood strain and coronary coronary heart price, which may be affected by stroke.

Understanding the area of the vagus nerve in stroke is important for developing new treatments and healing processes for stroke sufferers. By targeted on the vagus nerve, researchers can likely lessen contamination and decorate healing outcomes for stroke sufferers.

Overall, the vagus nerve plays a critical characteristic in stroke, and further research is wanted to completely understand its capability in stroke remedy and healing.

The Connection Between Vagus Nerve Stimulation and Stroke Recovery

The vagus nerve makes a amazing distinction in stroke recovery, and vagus nerve stimulation (VNS) has emerged as a capability treatment for stroke patients. VNS includes the use of a small device that is implanted within the neck and gives you electric impulses to the vagus nerve. These impulses can help to set off the brain's herbal healing mechanisms and promote recovery after a stroke.

Studies have confirmed that VNS can enhance motor feature, lessen infection, and decorate neuroplasticity in stroke patients. Neuroplasticity refers to the thoughts's capability to reorganize and shape new connections, that is essential for recuperation after a stroke. By stimulating the vagus nerve, VNS can help to decorate neuroplasticity and sell the growth of latest thoughts cells.

VNS has also been established to decorate cognitive feature in stroke sufferers. This is because the vagus nerve is installed to severa regions of the thoughts which are concerned in cognitive processing, which include the prefrontal cortex and the hippocampus. By stimulating the vagus nerve, VNS can help to beautify reminiscence, interest, and one-of-a-kind cognitive features that can be impaired after a stroke.

Overall, the connection between vagus nerve stimulation and stroke healing is a state-of-the-art place of studies. While more research are had to virtually recognize the advantages and risks of VNS for stroke patients, early effects recommend that this therapy may be a treasured addition to the equal antique treatments for stroke.

Clinical Trials and Research on Vagus Nerve Stimulation for Stroke

Clinical trials and studies on vagus nerve stimulation for stroke have verified thrilling outcomes. In a test posted in the magazine Stroke, researchers located that vagus nerve stimulation advanced motor function in stroke patients. The test worried 108 patients who had suffered a stroke and had been experiencing motor deficits. The sufferers had been randomly assigned to acquire both vagus nerve stimulation or a placebo remedy. After ninety days, the sufferers who acquired vagus nerve stimulation showed huge development in motor characteristic as compared to folks who acquired the placebo treatment.

Another observe posted within the mag Neuromodulation: Technology at the Neural

Interface located that vagus nerve stimulation advanced language function in stroke patients. The look at concerned seventeen sufferers who had suffered a stroke and had been experiencing language deficits. The patients received vagus nerve stimulation for 6 weeks and had been assessed for language feature in advance than and after the treatment. The effects confirmed that the sufferers had huge improvement in language function after the remedy.

These research propose that vagus nerve stimulation can be an powerful treatment for stroke sufferers who are experiencing motor or language deficits. However, more studies is wanted to absolutely understand the capability blessings and risks of vagus nerve stimulation for stroke. Clinical trials are presently underway to in addition take a look at using vagus nerve stimulation for stroke treatment.

Potential Risks and Side Effects of Vagus Nerve Stimulation for Stroke

While vagus nerve stimulation (VNS) has proven promise in stroke healing, it's miles vital to keep in thoughts the functionality dangers and aspect consequences related to this treatment.

One functionality danger of VNS is an infection at the internet site of the implant. This can upward push up if the incision net website isn't always well cared for or if the implant turns into dislodged. In a few cases, the implant can also want to be removed if the contamination is excessive.

Another chance is harm to the vagus nerve itself. This can stand up within the course of the implantation method or because of the electrical stimulation. Damage to the vagus nerve can bring about masses of signs and symptoms and symptoms, together with problem swallowing, hoarseness, and adjustments in heart charge.

In addition to the ones dangers, there also are potential component outcomes of VNS. These can embody nausea, vomiting, and dizziness.

Some patients also can enjoy adjustments in mood or conduct, which incorporates improved anxiety or irritability.

It is critical to word that no longer all sufferers will enjoy those dangers or issue consequences, and plenty of human beings have efficiently gone via VNS without any complications. However, it's miles critical to cautiously weigh the functionality dangers and benefits of this remedy in advance than you decide.

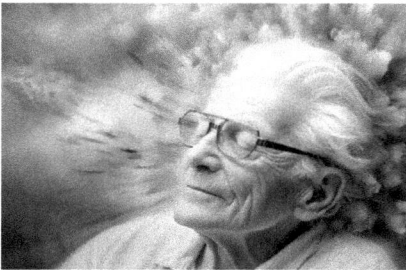

Vagus Nerve and Aging

Understanding the Role of the Vagus Nerve in Aging

As we age, our our our bodies undergo a multitude of modifications, every bodily and intellectual. One of the important issue players in this method is the vagus nerve.

Research has proven that the vagus nerve may also play a remarkable function inside the growing older technique. As we grow antique, the nerve can become a lot much less responsive, principal to pretty quite a number of age-related health issues. These can encompass cognitive decline, inflammation, and a weakened immune system.

However, trendy research have additionally recommended that stimulating the vagus nerve may additionally furthermore have a immoderate tremendous effect on those age-associated health situations. This has added about a growing hobby in the functionality of the vagus nerve as a device for selling wholesome getting old and sturdiness.

In this financial ruin, we're able to discover the area of the vagus nerve in developing older, and the way we're capable of harness its power to age gracefully. We will study the impact of vagus nerve stimulation on age-associated fitness situations, as well as the capability of the nerve to promote sturdiness. By facts the placement of the vagus nerve in developing older, we're able to take steps to optimize its feature and promote healthful getting old.

The Vagus Nerve and Age-Related Cognitive Decline

As we age, it is herbal to enjoy some degree of cognitive decline. However, studies has proven that the fitness of our vagus nerve may additionally play a key position in identifying the quantity of this decline.

The vagus nerve is accountable for regulating the parasympathetic anxious machine, that is responsible for rest. It additionally plays a role in regulating inflammation within the frame. When the vagus nerve is functioning optimally, it permits to sell healthful mind feature and cognitive abilties.

However, as we age, the vagus nerve can emerge as a whole lot tons less responsive, essential to a decline in cognitive feature. This decline can appear in pretty some techniques, which consist of reminiscence loss, trouble with trouble-fixing, and reduced hobby span.

Fortunately, there are steps we are able to take to help the health of our vagus nerve and possibly slow down age-associated cognitive decline. One of the satisfactory techniques to try this is thru regular exercise. Exercise has been verified to increase vagal tone, it really is a measure of the strength and responsiveness of the vagus nerve.

Other strategies for assisting vagus nerve health embody pressure discount strategies like meditation and deep respiration bodily sports activities, further to a healthful weight loss program wealthy in anti-inflammatory food like give up end result, vegetables, and omega-3 fatty acids.

By taking steps to assist the fitness of our vagus nerve, we are capable of doubtlessly slow down age-associated cognitive decline and keep our cognitive talents properly into our golden years.

The Impact of Vagus Nerve Stimulation on Age-Related Health Conditions

The vagus nerve performs a crucial role in regulating numerous physical abilties, such as coronary coronary coronary heart rate, digestion, and immune response. As we age, the functioning of the vagus nerve also can decline, essential to an entire lot of health situations. However, contemporary studies has proven that vagus nerve stimulation may additionally need to have a incredible impact on age-associated health conditions.

One of the most big benefits of vagus nerve stimulation is its functionality to decorate cognitive function in older adults. Studies have proven that stimulating the vagus nerve can beautify memory and hobby, in addition to lessen the risk of age-associated cognitive decline.

Vagus nerve stimulation has moreover been observed to be effective in treating quite a few age-associated fitness conditions, such as depression, tension, and persistent pain. The US Food and Drug Administration has permitted vagus nerve stimulation as a remedy for depression and epilepsy.

Additionally, vagus nerve stimulation has been established to have anti inflammatory results, which can be mainly useful for older adults who're extra prone to infection-related fitness situations which embody arthritis and cardiovascular disorder.

Overall, vagus nerve stimulation has the functionality to enhance the health and well-being of older adults. By harnessing the electricity of the vagus nerve, we will promote healthy growing vintage and decorate our superb of life in our later years.

The Role of the Vagus Nerve in Promoting Longevity

As we age, our our our our bodies undergo pretty some changes that can impact our everyday health and properly-being. One key thing that performs a function within the developing older approach is the vagus nerve.

Research has tested that the vagus nerve may additionally furthermore play a role in promoting durability. Studies have determined that humans with higher vagal tone – a degree of the electricity of the vagus nerve – usually generally generally tend to stay longer and function higher modern-day health consequences.

So how precisely does the vagus nerve promote durability? One key manner is through helping to alter infection within the frame. Chronic inflammation is a number one contributor to pretty quite a variety of age-related health situations, which consist of coronary coronary heart sickness, diabetes, and Alzheimer's disease. The vagus nerve lets in to maintain infection in test by using the usage of activating the frame's herbal anti-inflammatory response.

In addition, the vagus nerve may additionally additionally play a feature in promoting healthy developing older through using way of assisting the body's functionality to repair and regenerate cells. As we age, our cells end up a lot less inexperienced at repairing themselves, that can purpose more than a few fitness problems. By promoting cellular repair and regeneration, the vagus nerve may also assist to sluggish down the developing vintage way and keep us healthy for longer.

Chapter 8: Taking A Deep Breath Of Peace

1.1 THE BASICS: UNDERSTANDING BREATH AND THE VAGUS NERVE

Breathing is extra than in reality the easy act of bringing air into our lungs and letting it out. It's our body's manner of locating stability, especially at some stage in worrying times. The vagus nerve, a protracted nerve that connects the mind to many vital organs, plays a key function in this stability. When we breathe deeply, the vagus nerve sends indicators to our mind to reveal down the stress and flip up the relaxation. It's like telling your frame, "Hey, we have been given this. Let's lighten up."

Now, allow's get practical with some sports activities. We'll begin with the basics and drift to a few versions to hold topics sparkling and powerful.

Exercise 1-5: Basic Deep Breathing

Simple Deep Breathing:

Find a quiet spot.

Sit or lie down without issue.

Close your eyes, breathe in slowly via your nose for a bear in mind of four.

Hold for a rely of 4, then exhale for a consider of four.

Repeat for 5 minutes.

Counted Breath:

Similar to easy deep breathing, however this time enlarge your exhale to a rely of six.

Repeat for 5 minutes.

Belly Breathing:

Place one hand in your chest and the alternative on your belly.

Breathe in deeply via your nostril, letting your stomach push your hand out.

Exhale through pursed lips as if you had been whistling, experience the hand in your belly drift in, and use it to push all of the air out.

Repeat for five mins.

4-7-eight Breathing:

Inhale quietly via your nose for a count number wide variety of four.

Hold the breath for a recall of 7.

Exhale forcefully via your mouth for a rely of eight.

Repeat for 4 cycles.

Box Breathing:

Inhale for a remember of four, keep for a keep in thoughts of four.

Exhale for a keep in mind of four, and yet again preserve for a remember quantity of four.

Continue for five minutes.

Exercise 6-10: Seated Breathing Variations

Seated Side Stretch Breath:

While seated, inhale and stretch your palms overhead.

As you exhale, lean to the proper for a mild issue stretch. Inhale again to middle.

Exhale, leaning to the left. Continue for 5 mins.

Seated Twist Breath:

Inhale even as sitting tall, and as you exhale, twist to the proper, setting your left hand for your proper knee for a moderate twist.

Inhale once more to center, then exhale, twisting to the left. Continue for five mins.

Seated Forward Bend Breath:

Inhale sitting tall, exhale, and fold ahead lightly.

Inhale, rise lower back up, and repeat for five mins.

Seated Cat-Cow Breath:

Inhale, arching your lower back and looking up (that is the cow pose).

Exhale, rounding your once more and dropping your chin in your chest (this is the cat pose).

Continue for 5 mins.

Seated Heart Opener:

Sit at the threshold of your seat, clasp your arms at the back of your lower once more.

Inhale, lifting your chest and gently arching your decrease lower again.

Exhale, enjoyable another time to the start function. Continue for five minutes

Exercise 11-15: Standing Breathing Variations

Standing Side Stretch Breath:

Stand simply, inhale and stretch your fingers overhead.

As you exhale, lean to the right for a slight thing stretch. Inhale decrease again to middle.

Exhale, leaning to the left. Continue this for five mins.

Standing Forward Bend Breath:

Stand tall, inhale, and as you exhale, fold in advance from your hips, keeping a mild bend to your knees.

Inhale, slowly rolling lower back up to reputation.

Repeat for 5 minutes.

Standing Twist Breath:

Stand tall, inhale, and as you exhale, lightly twist your torso to the right.

Inhale again to middle, then exhale, twisting to the left.

Continue this for five mins.

Standing Backbend Breath:

Stand tall, area your palms for your decrease lower again for help.

Inhale, gently arching your again for a comfortable backbend. Exhale, returning to impartial.

Repeat for five mins.

Standing Mountain Breath:

Stand tall, feet grounded, fingers by means of your side.

Inhale, sweeping your hands overhead, searching up.

Exhale, bringing your palms back off with the aid of your component.

Continue this for five minutes.

Exercise 16-20: Movement-Integrated Breathing

Walk and Breathe:

Go for a walk. With every step, synchronize your breath. Inhale for 4 steps, hold for 4 steps, exhale for 4 steps.

Continue for a 10-minute stroll.

Stair Breathing:

Find a set of stairs. As you ascend, inhale for each step, and as you descend, exhale for every step.

Repeat for five minutes or as long as cushty.

Squat Breathing:

Stand with feet shoulder-width apart. Inhale as you decrease proper into a squat, exhale as you stand returned up.

Repeat for five minutes.

Lunge Breathing:

Stand tall, jump ahead right right into a lunge function as you inhale, pass back to popularity as you exhale.

Alternate legs and keep for five minutes.

Jumping Jack Breath:

Perform jumping jacks, inhaling as you jump out, exhaling as you leap in.

Continue for 5 mins or so long as comfortable.

1.2 GOING DEEPER: ADVANCED BREATHING EXERCISES

Exercise 21-25: Elevating the Basics

Extended Count Breath:

In a quiet spot, sit down down or lie down without troubles.

Inhale thru your nostril for a be counted of six, keep for a depend of six, and exhale for a be counted number variety of six.

Repeat this cycle for 5 minutes.

Double-Inhale Exhale:

Inhale two times via the nostril speedy, observed via an extended, controlled exhale through the mouth.

Repeat for 5 mins.

Breath Retention:

Inhale deeply through your nostril, preserve the breath for as long as comfortable.

Exhale slowly thru the mouth. Repeat for five mins.

Alternate Nostril Breathing:

Sit genuinely, close to your proper nostril together together with your right thumb, inhale via your left nostril.

Close your left nostril collectively with your ring finger, open your proper nose and exhale thru your proper nostril.

Continue this trade nose respiration for 5 minutes.

Ocean Breath (Ujjayi Pranayama):

Inhale deeply through your nostril, slightly constrict the again of your throat to create a slight "ocean" sound as you breathe.

Exhale thru your nose, preserving the equal constriction in your throat. Repeat for five mins.

Exercise 26-30: Integrating Movement

Breath with Arm Circles:

Stand or sit effortlessly. Begin circling your palms slowly at the same time as coordinating together along with your breath.

Inhale as your arms skip up and exhale as they arrive down. Continue for 5 mins.

Standing Forward Bend with Breath:

Stand tall, inhale and as you exhale, bend ahead out of your hips.

Inhale, come once more as plenty as reputation. Continue for five minutes.

Breath with Gentle Twists:

Seated or standing, inhale, and as you exhale, twist lightly to the proper.

Inhale lower back to center, exhale, twist lightly to the left. Continue for five minutes.

Breath with Side Bends:

Inhale, and as you exhale, bend gently to the right.

Inhale lower back to center, exhale, bend gently to the left. Continue for 5 minutes.

Walking Breath:

Go for a slight stroll. Inhale for 4 steps, keep for 4 steps, exhale for 4 steps. Continue for a ten-minute walk.

Exercise 31-35: Embracing Silence

Silent Breath Counting:

In a comfortable seated function, near your eyes and start to take a look at your natural breath.

Start counting your breaths silently, one count for each inhale and exhale.

Continue as a whole lot as a rely of 10, then begin lower lower lower back at one. Practice for five to 10 mins.

Observing the Pause:

In a quiet and snug spot, near your eyes.

Inhale deeply, and take a look at the slight pause in advance than you exhale. Exhale, and be conscious the pause earlier than your subsequent inhale.

Continue this observance for 5 mins.

Breath Awareness:

Sit or lie down without problem, final your eyes.

Simply study your breath, with out seeking to exchange it in any manner. Notice the temperature, tempo, and intensity.

Continue this remark for 5 minutes.

Listening to the Breath:

In a quiet place, near your eyes, loosen up and begin to pay attention to the sound of your breath.

Notice the sound of your inhale and exhale, and the silence in amongst. Continue for five mins.

Silent Breath Visualization:

Close your eyes, visualize the breath stepping into and leaving your frame.

Visualize calmness getting into with each inhale, and stress leaving with every exhale. Continue for five mins.

Exercise 36-forty: Expanding Horizons

Breath Expansion:

Inhale slowly and deeply via your nose, visualize filling your frame with breath out of your ft in your head.

Exhale, visualize the breath transferring out of your head proper right down to your ft. Continue for 5 minutes.

Ribcage Breathing:

Place your hands for your ribcage, sense it extend as you inhale, and settlement as you exhale.

Practice this for 5 minutes, feeling each movement of your ribs collectively along with your breath.

Back Body Breathing:

Lying for your once more, area your hands beneath your decrease lower lower back.

Try to press your hands together in conjunction with your again as you inhale, and enjoy the release as you exhale. Continue for 5 minutes.

Full Body Breath:

Lie down effects, start to inhale deeply, imagining your breath filling up your body from your toes in your head.

As you exhale, consider freeing all the anxiety from your head for your ft. Continue for five mins.

Expansive Breath:

In a comfortable seated position, on every inhale, envision your breath growing outward in all suggestions.

On each exhale, envision a moderate contraction inward. Continue this expansive respiratory for 5 minutes.

1.Three PAIRING BREATH WITH MOVEMENT

Exercise 41-forty five: Grounding Movements

Breath with Shoulder Rolls:

Sitting or reputation efficaciously, inhaling, rolling your shoulders up in the direction of your ears.

Exhale, rolling them decrease returned and down. Continue this round movement for 5 mins.

Breath with Neck Stretches:

Inhale, maintaining your neck right away, and as you exhale, lightly tilt your head to the right.

Inhale lower back to center, exhale, tilting to the left. Continue this mild movement for five minutes.

Breath with Arm Raises:

Stand or sit down down efficiently, inhale, raising your palms out to the edges and up overhead.

Exhale, bringing them backpedal through your components. Continue for five mins.

Breath with Seated Forward Folds:

Sitting effects with legs prolonged, inhale, sitting tall.

Exhale, folding beforehand gently from your hips. Inhale, coming lower again up. Continue for five minutes.

Breath with Side Bends:

Standing or sitting, inhale, and as you exhale, bend to the right, engaging in your right hand down toward the floor, left hand attaining over.

Inhale decrease once more to middle, exhale, bending to the left. Continue for 5 mins.

Exercise forty six-50: Energizing Movements

Breath with Standing Twists:

Standing without issues, inhale, and as you exhale, gently twist your torso to the right.

Inhale lower back to middle, exhale, twisting to the left. Continue this dynamic motion for five minutes.

Breath with High Knees:

Standing quite certainly, inhale, lifting your right knee, exhale, setting it down.

Inhale, lifting your left knee, exhale, placing it down. Continue for five mins.

Breath with Standing Forward Folds:

Standing tall, inhale, and as you exhale, fold beforehand out of your hips.

Chapter 9: Mindful Breathing

Exercise 51-fifty 5: Anchoring Awareness

Observing Breath:

Find a quiet location, sit down or lie down without problem, and close to your eyes.

Simply examine the glide of your breath with out converting it. Notice the chill of the inhale and heat of the exhale. Continue for five mins.

Counting Breath:

In a comfortable position, near your eyes, and begin counting your breaths backward from 10 to at least one, with each inhale and exhale.

If your mind drifts, lightly bring it once more to the very last variety you keep in mind. Continue for five mins.

Breath Focus:

Sit genuinely, close to your eyes, and location a hand in your stomach and the alternative to your chest.

Feel the rise and fall of every factor with the rhythm of your breath. Continue for five mins.

Sound of Breath:

In a serene spot, near your eyes, and turn your consciousness on the sound of your breath.

Let the slight rhythm lull your mind proper into a comfortable awareness. Continue for 5 minutes.

Breath Visualization:

Close your eyes and visualize a chilled scene with every inhale, and imagine freeing any anxiety with each exhale.

Continue this visualization for five mins.

Exercise 56-60: Deepening Mindful Connection

Breath and Body Scan:

Lie down with out problems, close to your eyes, and starting from your ft, frequently circulate your reputation up your frame to the crown of your head.

Notice any sensations as you breathe thru each element. Continue for 10 minutes.

Breath and Emotion:

Sit quietly, word how one-of-a-type emotions have an effect on your breath.

Name the emotion and look at with out judgment. Continue for five minutes.

Breath and Thought:

In a comfortable region, notice how your breath changes with exquisite thoughts.

Allow thoughts to move returned and bypass like clouds, continuously returning on your breath. Continue for 5 minutes.

Breath and External Sounds:

Find a quiet out of doors spot, close to your eyes, and be conscious the sounds around you.

Observe how your breath responds to excellent sounds. Continue for five minutes.

Breath and Gratitude:

With each inhale, bear in mind some element you are thankful for.

With each exhale, ship out thankfulness into the universe. Continue for 5 minutes.

1.Five TRACKING YOUR PROGRESS

Understanding the consequences of your respiratory practices is corresponding to having a verbal exchange with your self. It's a manner to pay attention to what your frame and thoughts are saying. Here are some simple techniques to song your improvement:

Observational Journaling:

Start a breathing exercise magazine. Each day, jot down the carrying sports activities you practiced and any most important results on your mood and strain levels. This isn't approximately critiquing your standard overall performance but noticing your critiques.

Breath Rate Monitoring:

Take take a look at of your breath fee earlier than and after your workout. Simply rely your breaths constant with minute. Over time, you will possibly have a look at a change in your breath charge which may be a trademark of advanced breath manipulate and probable, decreased pressure stages.

Mood Charting:

Create a mood chart. After each consultation, colour inside the day with a color that corresponds to the way you revel in. Over time, a sample might probable emerge displaying a correlation among your respiratory exercising and your moods.

Simple Check-ins:

Check in with yourself. How do you feel in advance than and after your respiration workout? Do you experience extra comfortable, targeted, or probable sleep comes less complicated? Your personal revel in is the remarkable gauge of improvement.

Digital Tools:

Utilize clean apps that may assist song your respiration practices, mood, and stress levels. There are severa free and paid apps to be had that provide an entire lot of monitoring talents.

Community Sharing:

If you are comfortable, share your testimonies with a depended on enterprise or network who moreover engage in respiration practices. Sharing and being attentive to others' tales can provide precious insights.

Congratulations for finishing the e-book's organising financial wreck. We have set out on a peaceful journey toward inner tranquility via our research of breath. We examined the significance of breathing, checked out more complex respiration techniques, connected breathing to interest, practiced aware breathing, and located the way to reveal our improvement. Every workout modified right into a step in the direction of perfecting the approach of calming one's respiration.

The emphasis will switch to the symbiotic interplay amongst physical exercising and the vagus nerve as we circulate into Chapter 2. But hold in mind that the expertise gained from this bankruptcy lays a sturdy foundation for what's to come back. The direction to serenity is sort of a river that meanders thru the landscapes of breath and bodily hobby, shifting slowly and frequently. So allow's carry the non violent breath rhythm into the exuberant dance of bodily exertion as we pass into the subsequent economic smash.

2.1 WARM-UP: PREPARING YOUR BODY

Exercise 61-70: Warm-up sports activities targeted on vagus nerve activation.

The act of warming up is not simply a training for the body but an invite for the vagus nerve to sign up for within the upcoming bodily hobby. A warmth-up is like knocking on the door in advance than moving into, a courteous gesture closer to your frame signaling the commencement of a physical endeavor.

Exercise 61-sixty five: Gentle Awakening

Neck Rolls:

Standing or sitting with out trouble, lightly roll your head in a round movement, feeling a slight stretch for your neck and shoulders. Continue for 3 minutes.

Shoulder Shrugs:

Lift your shoulders in the course of your ears on an inhale, and launch them down on an exhale. Continue this easy motion for three mins.

Arm Circles:

Extend your fingers out to the perimeters and perform sluggish, controlled round actions collectively along with your fingers, first forwards, then backwards. Continue for 3 mins.

Hip Circles:

Stand with toes hip-width aside, vicinity hands on hips, and make moderate spherical motions along with your hips. Continue for 3 minutes.

Knee Bends:

With ft shoulder-width aside, gently bend your knees as if you're approximately to sit down down lower back proper right into a chair, then straighten again up. Continue for three mins.

Exercise 66-70: Engaging the Breath

Breath-coordinated Squats:

Inhale as you decrease down proper into a squat, exhale as you stand once more up. Continue for 5 minutes.

Lunges with Breath:

Step ahead proper proper right into a lunge on an inhale, step lower back on an exhale. Alternate legs, preserve for five minutes.

Side Stretches with Breath:

Inhale as you stretch your arm overhead to at least one aspect, exhale as you come to center. Alternate facets, preserve for 5 minutes.

Forward Fold with Breath:

Inhale as you expand your spine, exhale as you fold forward out of your hips. Continue for five minutes.

Chapter 10: The Vagus Nerve And Exercise

Lie face down, fingers prolonged in the front of you. Lift your arms, chest, and legs off the floor as high as cushty. Hold for a few seconds, then lower. Repeat for 1-2 mins.

Exercise 76-80: Deepening the Connection

Leg Raises:

Lie for your decrease back, legs without delay. Lift legs up inside the direction of the ceiling, then lower backpedal without touching the ground. Continue for 1-2 minutes.

Reverse Crunches:

Lie on your returned, legs at a 90-diploma attitude. Lift hips off the ground, bringing knees within the route of chest. Lower back down. Continue for 1-2 mins.

Mountain Climbers:

Start in a push-up position, unexpectedly draw one knee into your chest, then transfer and convey the opposite knee into your chest, like walking in area. Continue for 1-2 minutes.

Boat Pose:

Sit on the floor, lean lower lower lower back, decorate legs, and enlarge arms beforehand. Hold for 30 seconds to at the least one minute, focusing for your breath.

V-Sit:

Lie lower lower back, fingers extended lower lower back. Lift legs and better frame at the equal time, forming a 'V' and reaching hands closer to toes. Lower back off. Continue for 1-2 minutes.

2.Three STRETCHING IT OUT

Exercise eighty one-ninety: Stretching carrying activities for rest and vagus nerve fitness.

Stretching is like extending a pleasing invitation to our vagus nerve to relax and partake in our bodily adventure within the path of calmness. Each stretch is an offering of peace, a pause in our day, a 2nd of calm amidst the storm of our busy lives.

Exercise 81-eighty 5: Gentle Eases

Neck Stretch:

Sit or stand successfully. Gently tilt your head to at the least one aspect, feeling a stretch along the problem of your neck. Hold for 30 seconds, then transfer sides.

Shoulder Stretch:

Bring your proper arm throughout your frame. Use your left hand to press your right arm closer to your chest until you experience a stretch at some stage in the outdoor of your shoulder. Hold for 30 seconds, then transfer aspects.

Triceps Stretch:

Reach your proper hand down the center of your lower returned, elbow pointing upwards. Gently keep your right elbow collectively collectively along with your left hand, feeling a stretch down your proper tricep and trouble frame. Hold for 30 seconds, then switch elements.

Cat-Cow Stretch:

On all fours, arch your decrease lower back up as you exhale (Cat), and dip it down as you inhale (Cow). Move fluidly amongst the ones positions for 1-2 mins.

Child's Pose:

From all fours, sit down down again onto your heels, accomplishing your arms out inside the the front or along your body. Rest proper right here, focusing in your breath for 1-2 mins.

Exercise 86-90: Deep Release

Spinal Twist:

Lie for your lower back, knees bent. Let your knees fall to 1 facet as you amplify your fingers out, keeping shoulders at the floor. Hold for 30 seconds to as a minimum one minute, then switch sides.

Puppy Pose:

From all fours, maintain hips over knees as you stroll your fingers out and reduce your chest towards the ground. Hold for 1-2 minutes.

Forward Fold:

Stand or take a seat, fold beforehand out of your hips, letting your head hang heavy. Hold for 1-2 minutes, allowing gravity to deepen the stretch.

Hip Flexor Stretch:

Step one foot forward right into a lunge, keeping the lower again knee on the floor. Gently press hips ahead to sense a stretch inside the the front of the back hip. Hold for 30 seconds, then transfer aspects.

Seated Forward Fold:

Sit on the floor, legs prolonged. Fold in advance from your hips, achieving inside the course of your ft. Hold for 1-2 mins.

2.Four YOGA AND THE VAGUS NERVE

Exercise ninety one-one hundred: Yoga poses and sequences for vagal stimulation.

Yoga is more than a bodily exercise; it's a quiet communique amongst your frame and your inner self, mediated by way of manner of manner of the vagus nerve. Each pose is a stanza on this silent communicate, every breath is a gentle beat that carries the rhythm of calm through the stretches and holds.

Exercise 91-90 5: Setting the Foundation

Mountain Pose (Tadasana):

Stand tall, feet collectively or hip-width apart. Engage your thighs, beautify your chest, and attain your arms overhead with arms managing each one among a kind. Breathe deeply, feeling the grounding strength thru your feet and the stretching thru your fingers.

Downward Dog (Adho Mukha Svanasana):

Start on all fours, tuck your ft, and lift your hips inside the course of the ceiling, forming an inverted 'V'. Stretch out through your legs and arms, respiratory deeply and feeling the lengthening for your spine.

Cat-Cow Pose (Marjarasana-Bitilasana):

On all fours, arch your back up as you exhale (Cat), and dip it down as you inhale (Cow). Move fluidly the various ones positions along side your breath for 1-2 mins.

Child's Pose (Balasana):

From all fours, sit again onto your heels, engaging in your arms out in front or along your body. Rest right here, focusing for your breath for 1-2 mins.

Cobra Pose (Bhujangasana):

Lie in your belly, fingers beneath your shoulders. Press through your arms to elevate your chest off the floor. Hold for a few breaths, then lower backtrack.

Exercise 96-one hundred: Flowing with Breath

Warrior I (Virabhadrasana I):

From reputation, step one foot decrease returned, maintaining the the the the front knee bent. Extend your hands overhead, fingers going through every particular. Breathe deeply and enjoy the strength to your legs and the stretch along your the front body.

Warrior II (Virabhadrasana II):

From Warrior I, open your hips and shoulders to stand sideways, extending your hands parallel to the ground. Look over your front hand and breathe deeply.

Triangle Pose (Trikonasana):

From Warrior II, straighten your the the front leg, acquire ahead, then tilt your torso, bringing your the front hand down to your shin or the floor, and the opportunity arm in the direction of the ceiling. Breathe deeply, feeling the hollow in your chest and aspect frame.

Seated Forward Fold (Paschimottanasana):

Sit on the floor, legs extended. Fold in advance out of your hips, carrying out towards your ft. Breathe deeply, feeling the stretch along your lower back.

Savasana (Corpse Pose):

- Lie flat on your once more, arms and legs prolonged, palms going through up. Close your eyes, breathe deeply, and permit your body to loosen up clearly. Stay on this pose for 5-10 mins, letting your breath sincerely stimulate the vagus nerve.

2.Five COOLING DOWN

Tips and physical sports for a groovy-down section.

Cooling down is like thanking your body for its tough art work and granting it the permission to relax. It's the duration in which the body transitions from the exertion of exercising to the kingdom of rest, and the vagus nerve plays a mild tune of rest, supporting us to ease into calmness.

Tip 1: Slow Transition

Don't rush thru the cool-down phase. As you finish your physical exercising, take a second to slow down your movements, frequently moving from immoderate electricity to a cushty country. This sluggish transition is useful for your coronary heart charge, your muscle groups, and your temper.

Walking it Off

A smooth and effective cool-down exercise is strolling. After your exercising, take a 5 to ten-minute stroll. This facilitates in bringing down the heart rate lightly, and it's additionally a high-quality manner to mirror to your exercising and revel in the serene aftermath of a top notch bodily exertion.

Tip 2: Stretching

Stretching is not best an exercising but a sign to the frame that it's time to lighten up. Stretching lets in in easing any tension inside the muscle companies, selling rest and preparing the body for rest.

136

Standing Forward Bend

Stand together with your ft hip-width aside, hinge at your hips and fold in advance, letting your head cling unfastened and your hands draw close or rest on the floor or your legs. This stretch permits in enjoyable the another time and neck muscle agencies, sending a relaxing sign through the vagus nerve.

Tip three: Hydration

Drinking water is a simple but effective way to assist the body transition from energetic to snug mode. It permits in flushing out any pollutants and rehydrating the frame.

Mindful Drinking

Take a tumbler of water, and as you drink, be aware about the feeling of the water, its temperature because it moves through your throat and into your stomach. This clean act of mindfulness can assist in triggering the relaxation reaction from the vagus nerve.

Tip 4: Deep Breathing

Just as we began out with breath, we near with it. Deep breathing is an instantaneous message to the vagus nerve to calm the body down.

Chapter 11: Breathe Awareness

Practice deep respiration sports, just like those in Chapter 1, focusing on the rhythm of your breath, and feeling the calmness unfold with each exhale.

Tip five: Reflect

Take a second to mirror in your workout, acknowledging the attempt and appreciating the adventure. This intellectual cool-down is as important due to the fact the physical one.

Journaling

Write down your reflections approximately the exercise, the manner you felt before, at some point of, and after, and any thoughts or observations that come to mind. This act of reflected picture can assist in tuning into your frame's responses and analyzing more approximately yourself.

Cooling down is an art work of transitioning, a slight bridge between the active and the restful. It's a workout that tells the vagus nerve, the body is ready to shift proper right into a rustic of calmness. And as you grasp this art work, you now not simplest emerge as attuned for your body's rhythms but moreover to the subtle whispers of the vagus nerve, guiding you softly toward a rustic of internal peace.

3HEALTHY EATING FOR VAGAL TONE

3.1 FUELING UP: FOODS THAT BOOST VAGAL TONE

Nutrition is a melodious song to which the vagus nerve dances gracefully. The components we consume play a pivotal position in how the vagus nerve plays, orchestrating a symphony of bodily competencies from digestion to mood regulation.

Tip 1: Colors on Your Plate

Variety is prime. Aim to fill your plate with a rainbow of colors from one-of-a-type quit end result and vegetables. These natural sunglasses frequently represent awesome vitamins and antioxidants, that are crucial for the maximum satisfying common performance of the vagus nerve.

Colorful Meal Planning

Let's plan regular with week's food making sure we include some of sunglasses in our eating regimen. For example, red tomatoes, inexperienced spinach, yellow bell peppers, purple eggplants, and so forth. Each meal have to have as a minimum 3 extraordinary colorings.

Tip 2: Omega-3 Fatty Acids

Omega-3 fatty acids are like best friends to the vagus nerve. They assist in lowering irritation and selling vagal tone.

Omega-three Rich Meal

Plan a meal rich in Omega-3 fatty acids. Some properly property encompass fatty fish like salmon, chia seeds, walnuts, and flaxseeds. Create a dish that incorporates one or greater of those assets.

Tip 3: Lean Proteins

Lean proteins aren't pleasant important for muscle restore and increase however moreover for the health of the vagus nerve. They provide the crucial amino acids which might be the constructing blocks of neurotransmitters managed via using the vagus nerve.

Protein-Packed Snacks

List down some protein-packed snacks you can have on the circulate. Include a combination of plant-primarily based actually and animal-based totally protein sources.

Tip four: Probiotics and Prebiotics

The gut is frequently called the second mind, and the vagus nerve is the line of communique between your gut and mind. Probiotics and prebiotics play a essential role in keeping a healthy intestine, which in turn helps the vagus nerve.

Fermented Foods

Incorporate fermented components wealthy in probiotics like yogurt, kefir, and sauerkraut into your food regimen. Plan a meal wherein a fermented meals is the well-known individual thing.

Tip five: Hydration

Again, water comes into play. Staying hydrated is critical for the smooth functioning of the vagus nerve.

Water Intake Tracker

Create a smooth water consumption tracker to make certain you're ingesting sufficient water at some degree within the day. Note down each glass of water you drink and purpose for at the least eight glasses an afternoon.

Feeding the body with the proper vitamins is like having a coronary coronary coronary heart-to-coronary heart with the vagus nerve, letting it apprehend you care. As we nourish ourselves with wholesome food, we gasoline the vagus nerve, empowering it to function at its incredible, creating a song a tune of fitness and harmony that resonates thru our entire being.

3.2 HYDRATION AND THE VAGUS NERVE

Water, the elixir of lifestyles, holds the reins in terms of the orchestration of bodily talents through the vagus nerve. Our body is sort of a river in which the currents of neurological signs go with the flow effortlessly even as properly-hydrated, however come across the rocks of disorder whilst dehydrated.

Tip 1: The 8x8 Rule

A easy rule to take into account is the 8x8 rule: 8 ounces.. Of water, eight times a day. It's easy to endure in mind and offers a number one guideline to ensure you're getting sufficient water.

Water Alarm

Set alarms in your telephone at particular intervals in the course of the day as a reminder to drink water. You also can use smart water bottles that remind you to stay hydrated.

Tip 2: Fruits and Veggies

Many cease end result and greens are water-wealthy and may contribute on your each day water intake. Cucumbers, watermelons, and oranges are excellent picks.

Hydration Salad

Create a salad the use of water-wealthy give up end result and vegetables. Note the smooth taste and the manner you experience after consuming it.

Tip three: Avoid Caffeine and Alcohol

While a tumbler of wine or a cup of coffee is enjoyable, those liquids can dehydrate you. It's advisable to restrict your consumption.

Beverage Swap

Try swapping one caffeinated beverage or alcoholic drink an afternoon with a pitcher of water or herbal tea and look at any adjustments in how you experience.

Tip four: Herbal Teas

Herbal teas are a fantastic way to stay hydrated and that they provide pretty various flavors to your flavor buds with none dehydrating results.

Herbal Exploration

Explore first rate natural teas and find out your favored. Note down how every one makes you enjoy.

Tip five: Check Your Urine

The coloration of your urine is a honest indicator of your hydration degree. Aim for a mild, faded colour which shows correct hydration.

Urine Color Log

Keep a log of the coloration of your urine for each week to better understand your hydration levels and modify your water intake therefore.

The voyage of water from the tip of your lips right all the way down to the mobile degree is a terrific journey that holds the promise of strength, clarity, and a harmonious speak the various intestine and the thoughts via the vagus nerve. As every droplet descends, wearing with it the essence of lifestyles, the vagus nerve hums a track of approval, orchestrating a dance of molecules that invigorates every mobile, each tissue, and each organ. The simplicity of hydration, an act so smooth however profoundly impactful, paves the way for a extra healthy, more colorful existence.

three.Three MINDFUL EATING

Mindful consuming is like having a coronary coronary heart-to-coronary coronary heart in conjunction with your food. It's about appreciating the colours, textures, and flavors in your plate, while being attentive to the cues from your body approximately hunger and fullness. This exercising can notably have an impact at the vagus nerve, enhancing its feature and eventually, promoting a state of calm and satisfaction.

Tip 1: Chew Slowly

Chewing is step one in the digestive manner, and doing it slowly can help in higher digestion and absorption of vitamins.

Chew Count

In your subsequent meal, depend how generally you chunk every bite. Aim for at the least 30 chews in advance than swallowing.

Chapter 12: Review And Revise

At the prevent of the week, assessment your meal plan. What worked? What didn't? Adjust your plan for the subsequent week based to your observations.

Meal planning is like having a talk with yourself about your dietary desires and goals. It's about placing yourself up for achievement in a way that feels precise and is sustainable. And in this speak, your vagus nerve has a voice too, guiding you closer to alternatives that foster a feel of calm and nicely-being.

Three.5 SUPPLEMENTATION

Supplements can be an wonderful nice friend in nurturing your vagus nerve, in particular while your every day food fall short of the preferred vitamins. However, it's miles crucial to tread this path with a knowledgeable thoughts, know-how what dietary dietary supplements can assist and the manner to consist of them for your diet with out going overboard.

Tip 1: Omega-three Fatty Acids

Omega-3 fatty acids are stated for their anti inflammatory houses that might, in turn, useful resource vagal fitness.

Omega-three Journal

Track your omega-3 consumption via food and nutritional supplements for every week. Notice any modifications in your mood and physical sensations.

Tip 2: Probiotics

A healthful gut is a playground for the vagus nerve. Probiotics can help preserve a nice surroundings in your intestine.

Probiotic Exploration

Try a probiotic complement for a month, and examine any adjustments to your digestion and stylish feeling of calm.

Tip three: Vitamin B12

Vitamin B12 is vital for nerve fitness. It's like a bit cheerleader to your vagus nerve, preserving it in suitable spirits.

B12 Tracker

Monitor your Vitamin B12 stages through meals and dietary dietary supplements. Consult with a healthcare issuer to make sure you're getting an true sufficient amount.

Tip 4: Magnesium

Magnesium is kind of a spa day for your vagus nerve, assisting it loosen up and characteristic easily.

Magnesium Moments

Include a magnesium supplement on your ordinary and word if your sleep exquisite improves over time.

Tip five: Vitamin D

Sunshine food plan, Vitamin D, isn't always quite plenty bone health, but it's a chum of your vagus nerve too.

Sunshine and Supplement

Track your Vitamin D consumption thru sunshine, food, and dietary dietary supplements. Aim for at the least 20 minutes of daylight hours publicity every day.

Tip 6: Herbal Helpers

Certain herbs like Ashwagandha and Rhodiola may be supportive of your vagus nerve.

Herbal Diary

Try an natural complement seemed for assisting nerve fitness, and maintain a diary of any adjustments you study in your temper and pressure levels.

Tip 7: Consult a Professional

Before at the side of any complement in your recurring, it's sensible to speak approximately with a healthcare professional.

Professional Guidance

Schedule a consultation with a nutritionist or a healthcare issuer to talk about your supplement plan, making sure it aligns at the side of your health goals and is supportive of your vagus nerve.

Supplementation can be a strong bridge between your each day diet and the nutritional haven your vagus nerve craves. It's about filling within the gaps at the identical time as making sure a harmonious dating among your meals and dietary dietary supplements. As we near this chapter on vitamins, we've equipped ourselves with a basket whole of expertise on how to fuel our frame to choose the vagus nerve, developing a ripple of calmness in our inner ocean.

MEDITATION AND AWARENESS

Congrats on crusing via the number one 3 chapters of this journey towards a calmer self! You've laid a robust foundation with the useful resource of manner of facts the area of respiratory, bodily pastime, and vitamins in nurturing your vagus nerve. You've explored a plethora of wearing sports and accumulated an arsenal of know-how on a manner to keep your vagus nerve glad. You're no longer certainly analyzing a e-book; you are evolving with each net web web page you switch.

4.1 GROUNDING TECHNIQUES

Grounding is like telling your frame, "Hey, I'm right right here, I'm gift." It's about connecting to the right here and now, that may be a wonderful way to coax your vagus nerve proper into a kingdom of relaxation. Let's dive into some sporting occasions that can help you get grounded and stimulate your vagus nerve.

Exercise one 0 one: Five Senses Exercise

Sit effects.

List five topics you may see, 4 subjects you may contact, three subjects you can pay interest, 2 subjects you could odor, and 1 thing you can taste. It's about immersing your self inside the gift 2d.

Exercise 102: Earth Touch

Stand barefoot on the floor. Feel the earth beneath your ft.

Visualize roots growing out of your ft into the earth, anchoring you. Take ten deep breaths.

Exercise 103: Muscle Tensing and Releasing

Start collectively along with your feet and paintings your way up on your head.

Tense each muscle enterprise for some seconds, then release.

Exercise 104: Mindful Walking

Walk slowly and deliberately.

Feel the sensation in your legs and ft with each step.

Exercise a hundred and five: Stone Grounding

Hold a stone or a crystal.

Focus on its texture, temperature, and weight. Close your eyes and take ten deep breaths.

Exercise 106: Breath Awareness

Sit quite honestly.

Focus on your breath. Feel the cool air as you breathe in and the fine and comfortable air as you breathe out.

Exercise 107: Color Grounding

Choose a colour.

Look round and word everything round you of that coloration.

Exercise 108: Tree Pose (Vrksasana)

Stand on one leg.

Place the possibility foot at the internal thigh of the reputation leg, like a tree. Hold for a minute.

Exercise 109: Guided Imager

Close your eyes.

Visualize a serene location, feel the calmness seep into each mobile of your frame.

Exercise a hundred and ten: Mindful Eating

Eat a small snack.

Chew slowly, savoring every flavor and texture.

These wearing sports are your toolkit for grounding. They're like a moderate nudge to your vagus nerve pronouncing, "Hey, it's safe, you may lighten up." Grounding is an invite to the prevailing 2nd, a location wherein your vagus nerve can breathe a sigh of comfort. The splendor of grounding is its simplicity. It's a smooth whisper to the chaos of each day life saying, "Shhh, relax."

four.2 MINDFULNESS MEDITATION

As we tread in addition into the coronary coronary heart of mindfulness, meditation simply unveils itself as a powerful excellent buddy. Mindfulness meditation isn't always about escaping truth, but as an opportunity immersing ourselves in the present 2d, with a mild curiosity and beauty. It's like saying to your self, "Hey, some factor is taking region right now, it's good enough. I'm right here for it." And bet what? Your vagus nerve is all ears, organized to soak in the calmness that mindfulness meditation can deliver. Let's delve into some practices with a purpose to allow you to domesticate this serene u . S . A . Of thoughts.

Exercise 111: Breath Awareness Meditation

Find a quiet spot.

Close your eyes, and bring your attention in your breath. Notice the rhythm, the sensation of air flowing outside and inside. Whenever your thoughts drifts, gently bring it lower back on your breath.

Chapter 13: Guided Meditations

Venturing similarly into the sector of meditation, guided meditations surface as a pleasant associate in this voyage. They are similar to the slight hand of a guide, main you via the dense wooded area of your mind, helping you navigate through the underbrush to discover clearings of calm and perception. Your vagus nerve too, responds to this steering, tuning into the rhythms of relaxation and peace that the ones practices can provide. Let's discover some guided meditations tailor-made to foster a hearty connection with our vagus nerve.

Exercise 121: Guided Breathing Meditation

Find a guided respiratory meditation online or via a meditation app.

Follow the voice guiding you, as you attention for your breath, feeling the calming consequences ripple via you.

Exercise 122: Progressive Muscle Relaxation

Seek a guided revolutionary muscle rest recording.

Follow along, tensing and then thrilling every muscle group as directed, melting away anxiety from head to toe.

Exercise 123: Guided Visualization

Pick a guided visualization meditation that appeals to you.

Let the narrative supply you to serene places, as you visualize calming scenes, feeling a enjoy of peace envelop you.

Exercise 124: Guided Mindfulness Meditation

Locate a mindfulness meditation guide that resonates with you.

Allow the guide to walk you through the stairs of grounding yourself in the gift 2nd, noticing the whole lot with a slight, non-judgmental attention.

Exercise 100 twenty five: Yoga Nidra Meditation

Find a guided Yoga Nidra session.

Follow the instructions, diving right into a deep country of rest on the identical time as final aware.

Exercise 126: Guided Loving-Kindness Meditation

Choose a loving-kindness meditation manual.

Repeat the declaring phrases, extending love and pinnacle wants to yourself and others.

Exercise 127: Chakra Balancing Meditation

Seek a guided chakra meditation.

Follow along as you visualize recuperation electricity moving thru your frame's energy centers, fostering a experience of stability and harmony.

Exercise 128: Guided Sleep Meditation

Pick a sleep meditation guide for a restful night time's sleep.

Let the soothing voice and narrative lull you proper into a deep, restorative sleep.

Exercise 129: Guided Nature Meditation

Select a nature-primarily based genuinely guided meditation.

Visualize the scenes defined, feeling a deep reference to the natural international.

Exercise one hundred thirty: Guided Journaling Meditation

Locate a guided journaling meditation that activates introspection.

Follow alongside, writing down your thoughts and insights as added approximately via the use of the usage of the guide.

Guided meditations provide a based pathway into the nation-states of internal calm, rest, and self-exploration. They are your accomplice, your guide, via the meditative adventure, making the exploration both to be had and fun. As you take a look at the guiding voice, you're not by myself; your vagus nerve is right there with you, relishing inside the tranquility and revel in of ease that the ones practices convey in.

four.4 PROGRESSIVE RELAXATION

Progressive rest is like whispering candy nothings in your muscle businesses, coaxing them into a country of utter rest, one enterprise at a time. It's much like having a slight communication together along with your body, acknowledging the tension it holds, after which granting it permission to permit that anxiety waft. This soothing talk now not handiest calms the muscle mass however moreover sends waves of tranquility along the pathways of your vagus nerve. Let's delve into a few carrying activities that assist in orchestrating this serene talk amongst thoughts, frame, and vagus nerve.

Exercise 131: Forehead Relaxation

Sit or lie down in a comfy function.

Focus in your forehead. Imagine it smoothing out as though a warm temperature, clean cloth is gently wiping away any furrows.

Breathe deeply, feeling the gain seep into your brow.

Exercise 132: Jaw Easing

Maintain your comfortable function.

Now shift your attention on your jaw. Let it float slack, developing vicinity amongst your pinnacle and decrease enamel.

Enjoy the sensation of release as you breathe inside and outside.

Exercise 133: Shoulder Drop

Still in your relaxed spot, draw your interest on your shoulders.

With every exhale, allow them to drop far from your ears, feeling the anxiety melting away.

Exercise 134: Arm and Hand Release

Extend your cognizance all the way right right down to your hands and arms.

Let them broaden heavy and snug, imagining any tension dripping off your fingertips.

Exercise one hundred thirty 5: Back Relaxation

Now, visualize a wave of rest starting from the top of your backbone, trickling down vertebrae with the aid of vertebrae, all of the manner in your lower decrease again.

Feel your lower back sinking into the assist under, steady and comfortable.

Exercise 136: Hip and Seat Softening

Let this wave of rest waft in addition all the way right down to your hips and seat.

Feel them soften and yield to the pull of gravity.

Exercise 137: Leg and Foot Ease

Continue this soothing wave down your legs, all the manner on your feet.

Imagine any final anxiety flowing out thru your feet, leaving your body.

Exercise 138: Full-Body Scan

Now, do a moderate test from the crown of your head to the suggestions of your feet, acknowledging any spots of hysteria.

Send your breath to those spots, ushering in relaxation.

Exercise 139: Breath Awareness

Turn your cognizance inward to your breath, feeling the cool air as you inhale and the first-rate and cushty air as you exhale.

Let your breath be the anchor that holds you in this nation of deep relaxation.

Exercise one hundred forty: Vagal Tone Visualization

In this kingdom of tranquility, visualize your vagus nerve as a non violent, gentle river, flowing with out problem through your body.

With every breath, believe this river developing clearer and extra serene, signifying a balanced and sturdy vagal tone.

four.Five TRACKING YOUR MINDFULNESS JOURNEY

As we unfurled the petals of mindfulness, we positioned a quiet sanctuary inner, an area in which the vagus nerve too determined its rhythm of calm. But how can we bear in mind the perfume of peace in a worldwide that regularly smells of hurry? Tracking our mindfulness journey isn't about marking a tick list; it's approximately capturing the essence of every silent second spent in introspection, each slight be privy to calm that touched the coronary heart. It's about seeing the mirrored picture of our inner sky in the nevertheless waters of awareness. This subtle artwork of monitoring isn't a inflexible shape but a fluid dance that actions with the rhythm of our studies. Here are some approaches to preserve the moments of mindfulness lightly within the hands of our hobby.

Mindfulness Journaling: A magazine isn't handiest a ebook; it's a replicate reflecting our inner world. Each internet page holds the whispers of our soul, the subtle shifts in our being as we delve deeper into the exercise of mindfulness. The act of penning down our evaluations, the texture of silence, the palette of emotions, and the dialogues with the self, crafts a pathway of popularity. It's like having a conversation with our inner being, a speak that's slight, honest, and illuminating.

Mood Tracker: Our moods are like colours portray the canvas of our day. Some days are blue with calm, others may be pink with rush. A temper tracker is a clean but insightful way to peer the shades of our inner sky. It's charming to have a examine how the palette brightens as we nestle into the exercise of mindfulness, how the colors dance to the track of a soothed vagus nerve.

Breathing Patterns: Our breath is the slight tide that washes the seashores of silence. Tracking our respiration styles before and after meditation can spread a tale of calm. It's a story knowledgeable with the useful aid of the rhythm of our breath, of approaches the waves of hurry recede and the shorelines of stillness amplify.

Meditation Timer: The mild chime marking the start and cease of our meditation practice is kind of a smooth embody of time. It holds the distance for us to dive inward, to the touch the geographical regions of silence and stillness. A meditation timer is a humble partner on this inward adventure, anchoring us inside the gift.

Mindfulness Apps: In a worldwide that's virtual, why now not have a pocket accomplice to remind us of the course of calm? Mindfulness apps are like gentle reminders amidst the noise, nudging us to pause, breathe, and dive inward.

Body Scan Record: The frame is a vessel preserving the memories of our tales. A positioned up-meditation body check is like studying the ones recollections, information the language of our muscle companies and bones. Noticing the areas of relaxation and tension is an insightful narrative of the manner mindfulness is weaving its magic.

Vagal Tone Check: Our vagus nerve is form of a gentle vine, its health reflecting the satisfactory of our mindfulness exercise. A everyday test on our vagal tone may be an inspiring feedback, a sworn statement to the stunning adjustments blooming internal.

Sharing Circles: Sharing our journey with others strolling the equal course of mindfulness is like weaving a tapestry of memories. Each thread holds a tale, a mastering, a 2nd of focus. Sharing circles are a region of collective mirrored image, a garden in which the seeds of belief blossom via shared recollections.

Wow, have a observe how far you have journeyed thru the tapestry of this e book. It's like a tranquil river you've got been rowing your boat on, each bankruptcy a stretch of waters explored, along with your oars of interest stirring the depths. Through four chapters, you have navigated via the geographical regions of breath, frame, vitamins, and the calming seashores of mindfulness. You've no longer in fact have a look at; you've got engaged, practiced, and perhaps begun to feel a serene ripple thru your being. It's lovable, is not it? The manner phrases on paper have the strength to guide actual transformation within.

Now, as we steer our boat into the sunrise of Chapter five, the waters in advance gleam with the promise of every day workout routines that echo with the rhythm of vagal health. As the number one rays of morning kiss the earth, there may be a sweet invitation within the air to start the day with easy gestures of care. It's a call to which our vagus nerve responds with a clean hum of readiness.

Morning Routines:

The morning is kind of a easy canvas, and our sporting sports are the strokes of coloration that set the tone for the day. Each movement, each desire is a brushstroke at the canvas. The morning exercise routines aren't inflexible schedules; they'll be mild rhythms, an intuitive dance with the dawn.

Exercise 141-one hundred and fifty: Morning carrying sports for a day of calm:

As the morning sun casts a golden glow, it's time to shake off the night time time time's stillness and invite a calm strength into our body and mind. These sporting occasions are mild whispers to our vagus nerve, announcing, "Wake up, it's a ultra-modern day."

Sun Salutations: As the selection shows, it's a warmth greeting to the solar, a chain of actions that reach and awaken every a part of our frame. The beauty of Sun Salutations lies in its simplicity and waft, a choreography of care that prepares us for the day.

Breath Awareness: The day starts with the number one aware breath. Seated efficiently, we've a take a look at the mild ebb and drift of our breath, feeling its coolness because it enters, and its warm temperature because it leaves.

Gentle Neck Stretches: Our neck is home to the vagus nerve, and moderate stretches can whisper a clean be-careful call to it. Simple tilts and rotations of the neck are like announcing perfect morning to our inner calm.

Shoulder Rolls: The smooth act of rolling our shoulders can shake off any stiffness, making location for ease and luxury as we step into the day.

Leg Shakes: A playful shake of every leg, letting loose, shaking off the vintage, and making region for the present day day's strength.

Toe Tapping: A rhythmical tapping of our ft, a easy song to which our day begins, activating the lower part of our frame.

Mindful Sipping: A warmth cup of natural tea or water, sipped slowly, tasting the essence of morning calm.

Gratitude Journaling: Penning down 3 topics we're grateful for, it's a mild gaze at the benefits that color our life.

Nature Walk: A short walk amidst nature, the trees, the chirping birds, it's a sweet serenade to our senses, a way to ground ourselves.

Vagal Massage: A moderate rubdown alongside the neck, a easy touch that echoes thru the vagus nerve, putting a tone of calm.

Chapter 14: Routines For A Vagal Healthy Life

five.1 MORNING ROUTINES

Wow, have a have a look at how a long way you've got journeyed thru the tapestry of this e-book. It's like a tranquil river you've been rowing your boat on, every chapter a stretch of waters explored, together together with your oars of curiosity stirring the depths. Through 4 chapters, you've got navigated via the geographical regions of breath, frame, vitamins, and the calming beaches of mindfulness. You've not certainly check; you've got engaged, practiced, and possibly started out out to experience a serene ripple thru your being. It's lovable, is not it? The manner terms on paper have the electricity to manual real transformation interior.

Now, as we steer our boat into the sunrise of Chapter five, the waters earlier gleam with the promise of daily physical video games that echo with the rhythm of vagal health. As the number one rays of morning kiss the earth, there can be a sweet invitation within the air to start the day with smooth gestures of care. It's a name to which our vagus nerve responds with a easy hum of readiness.

Morning Routines:

The morning is form of a smooth canvas, and our exercises are the strokes of coloration that set the tone for the day. Each movement, each desire is a brushstroke at the canvas. The morning carrying occasions aren't inflexible schedules; they're moderate rhythms, an intuitive dance with the dawn.

Exercise 141-100 and fifty: Morning carrying activities for an afternoon of calm:

As the morning sun casts a golden glow, it's time to shake off the night time time time's stillness and invite a peaceful energy into our frame and thoughts. These wearing sports are gentle whispers to our vagus nerve, pronouncing, "Wake up, it's a present day day."

1.   Sun   Salutations: As   the   decision
suggests, it's a warm temperature greeting to
the sun, a sequence of actions that reach and
awaken each part of our body. The splendor
of Sun Salutations lies in its simplicity and go
together with the float, a choreography of
care that prepares us for the day.

2.   Breath   Awareness: The   day   begins
offevolved   offevolved   with   the   primary
conscious breath. Seated pretty without a
doubt, we test the clean ebb and drift of our
breath, feeling its coolness because it enters,
and its warm temperature as it leaves.

3.   Gentle Neck Stretches: Our neck is
domestic to the vagus nerve, and mild
stretches can whisper a smooth be-careful
call to it. Simple tilts and rotations of the neck
are like saying particular morning to our
internal calm.

four. Shoulder Rolls: The smooth act of
rolling our shoulders can shake off any
stiffness, making region for ease and luxury as
we step into the day.

five.   Leg Shakes: A playful shake of each leg, letting free, shaking off the antique, and making region for the contemporary day's strength.

6.   Toe Tapping: A rhythmical tapping of our ft, a smooth track to which our day starts offevolved, activating the lower a part of our body.

7.   Mindful Sipping: A warm temperature cup of natural tea or water, sipped slowly, tasting the essence of morning calm.

eight. Gratitude Journaling: Penning down 3 subjects we're grateful for, it's a mild gaze at the advantages that shade our lifestyles.

nine. Nature Walk: A short stroll amidst nature, the timber, the chirping birds, it's a candy serenade to our senses, a manner to ground ourselves.

10.   Vagal Massage: A mild massage alongside the neck, a gentle contact that echoes through the vagus nerve, setting a tone of calm.

five.2 MIDDAY RESETS

As the sun climbs higher inside the sky, marking the midday, it's far a mild reminder to pause, breathe, and realign. It's so smooth to get caught up inside the whirlwind of the day, the limitless to-dos, the ticking clock. Yet, our vagus nerve craves the ones moments of stillness amidst the hustle. The midday reset isn't about halting the day's momentum; it's far about superb-tuning it, ensuring the melody of our day continues in harmony with our inner rhythm.

Midday Resets:

The concept of a midday reset is much like a quick retreat, a smooth oasis within the wilderness of each day chores. It's not about carving out hours; it's about sparing a couple of minutes to go back domestic to ourselves, to the touch the silence that dwells internal, even amidst the day's noise.

Exercise 151-one hundred sixty: Quick carrying occasions to reset and stimulate the vagus nerve:

Even a smooth pause can be transformative. The bodily video games said under are mild nudges, a easy call to our vagus nerve, reminding it to preserve singing the tune of calm.

1. Mindful Breathing: Finding a quiet spot, we sit down and near our eyes, tuning into the rhythm of our breath. It's a easy yet profound manner to track out the noise and song into our inner calm.

2. Neck Stretch: A moderate tilt of the neck to and fro, a tender stretch that speaks right now to the vagus nerve, liberating any anxiety dwelling there.

three. Shoulder Shrug: A slight shrug of the shoulders, a clean movement that helps shake off any weight we had been sporting.

four. Humming: The easy hum resonates thru our body, a sweet music that the vagus nerve responds to.

5. Hydration: Sipping water, a reminder to live hydrated, a smooth however crucial word in the melody of our fitness.

6. Walking: A brief walk, every step a meditation, each breath a prayer. It's a mild movement that permits spoil the monotony of the day.

7. Yawn and Stretch: The maximum herbal reset button - an first-rate yawn discovered through a slight stretch, a candy invitation to lighten up.

eight. Guided Relaxation: A brief guided relaxation audio, a soft voyage into tranquility even amidst a busy day.

nine. Healthy Snack: A second to nourish our body with a healthful snack, a reminder of the candy interaction amongst vitamins and nerve fitness.

10. Gratitude Reminder: A second to mirror on one detail that's going properly nowadays, a candy pause that fills our being with a gentle glow of gratitude.

These carrying occasions are not a checklist, however a buffet, providing terrific flavors of reset. You can select one or some, based at the rhythm of your day. It's approximately locating what resonates with you, what lets in you return domestic to that location of calm and clarity, even amidst the day's dance.

five.Three EVENING WIND-DOWN

As the day begins to fold into the moderate shades of nighttime, it's miles a name to slowly wind down, to transition from the day's hustle to the tranquil embody of the night time. The middle of the night wind-down is a slight bridge between the lively and the restorative, a candy serenade to our vagus nerve, permitting it to waft right into a rustic of calm due to the fact the arena round us begins to quieten.

Chapter 15: Good Sleep Practices

Tips and sports to beautify vagus nerve feature and sleep

Sleep isn't clearly a pause in our each day normal; it's a deep dive into the frame's innate potential to heal and restore itself. The wonderful of sleep profoundly impacts how the vagus nerve abilties, placing the tone for the manner we navigate the demanding situations of the upcoming day. Here's the manner to foster a friendship between proper sleep practices and your vagus nerve:

1.   Establish a Ritual: Like a mild lullaby, a pre-sleep ritual tells your frame it's time to transition into relaxation. This can be a smooth routine of light studying, slight stretching, or soothing track.

2.   Unplug: The global can wait. It's essential to unplug from digital gadgets at least an hour in advance than sleep, providing a smash from the constant stimulation and allowing the vagus nerve to ease into its night time time-time function.

3.   Darkness is Your Ally: A dark, cool room is an invitation for deep sleep. It's a sign up your mind to release melatonin, the hormone that encourages sleep, supporting the vagus nerve in transitioning your frame into a rustic of rest.

four. Mind Your Diet: A light dinner, preferably multiple hours before bedtime, guarantees your digestive device isn't overtaxed as you try to sleep, permitting the vagus nerve to cognizance on restorative techniques.

five. Calm Your Mind: A whirlpool of thoughts can keep away from the exceptional of sleep. Techniques like meditation or smooth respiratory bodily games can assist calm the thoughts, placing the extent for the vagus nerve to function optimally.

www.ingramcontent.com/pod-product-compliance
Lightning Source LLC
Chambersburg PA
CBHW051728020426
42333CB00014B/1215